"Hearing Loss Help" is an effective patient education book. Simple, easy to read and understand, it is the first popular book which addresses the needs and problems of a very large number of people—those with beginning or mild hearing losses **and** the 'others' in their lives.

"I provide it to all my patients and 'insist' they read it before the next appointment. They learn far more from reading the book at home than I can teach them (or they can remember) during the limited time we have together. And, when they return, we have ample time to talk about any questions they may have about their particular problems.

"I congratulate Alec Combs on his accomplishment. Read and think about what he has to say—it may be very important in your life."

D.E. Regan, Ph.D.
Audiologist

"I saw your book in my library and wanted one for someone very dear to me."

P.A., Paramus, New Jersey

"Yesterday, I found your book at the public library. I couldn't put it down. The title couldn't be more appropriate. I am enclosing a money order for my own copy."

L.G., Goldsboro, North Carolina

"This book has become a major tool in my practice. When 'important others' are encouraged to help in advance, my work is much easier and hearing aids are nearly always accepted.

"Alec Combs comes through as a compassionate writer. One patient with a beginning hearing loss said after reading the book, 'He must be a kind man.'"

Stephanie E. Moss, M.A.
Audiologist and Hearing Aid Dispenser

HEARING
LOSS
HELP

How you *can help someone with a hearing loss . . . and how* they *can help themselves*

Alec Combs

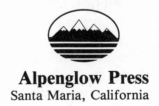

Alpenglow Press
Santa Maria, California

HEARING LOSS HELP
by Alec Combs

Published by:
Alpenglow Press
Post Office Box 1841
Santa Maria, CA 93456 U.S.A.

Extreme care has been used in researching and writing this book accurately, but no responsibility can be assumed for any errors or omissions. It is the responsibility of each reader to exercise good judgment in using any suggestions herein. And in no instance is anything herein intended to replace proper medical care and advice.

Library of Congress Cataloging-in-Publication Data:
Combs, Alec, 1918-
     Hearing loss help.

     Bibliography: p.
     Includes index.
     1. Hearing disorders—Popular works. 2. Deafness —Popular works. 3. Hearing aids. I. Title.
RF290.C66 1986   617.8'9   86-1135
ISBN 0-935997-14-8 (pbk.)

This book is dedicated to Grace
. . . who graces my life these days,

and to all those important others
who help us as we struggle in a
world designed for people with
normal hearing.

ACKNOWLEDGMENTS and CREDITS

My gratitude to the many people who, over a long period of time, had a part in shaping the contents of this book.

My warmest personal thanks to these people in particular who had a more direct part:

Mindy Bingham (author, publisher)
Doris Bryant, M.A. (psychology)
Bobbie Lee Garrett, M.A. (audiology)
Victor P. Garwood, Ph.D. (audiology)
Thomas Gordon, Ph.D. (psychology)
Stanley Hawks, M.S. (physics)
R.A. Hendricks, M.D. (medical)
Chelle Hendrix (book design)
John and Ginny Moore (friends . . . and more)
Stephanie Moss, M.A. (audiology)
George Mulder, Ph.D. (psychology)
Mike Noll (photography)
Dan Poynter (author, publisher)
and to Terri Pinckard
who showed the way

Cover by Robert Howard

FOREWORD

I have known Alec Combs for many years—as a person and as a student in my psychology classes.

He has lived a full and interesting life, a life of wide experiences, of ups and downs, but far more achievements than disappointments. I don't know of anyone more appropriate or capable of writing this book.

When Alec approached me about writing the foreword for his book, I felt honored and accepted even while knowing full well I was already far overloaded with work. The last thing I needed was to review another book. But I knew Alec and wanted to see what he had done. And almost immediately he had my attention.

The quirks of life continually amaze me: here comes his manuscript and it seemed he was writing directly to me. It was almost as if he'd been living in our home and knew what was happening to *me*. I had all the early warning signs he describes and my way of life *had* slowly changed.

I was aware of not hearing quite as well, but I hadn't connected this fact with the frustrations hearing loss was causing me (and human behavior is my work). I sat and thought into the night about my situation and about how many others across this country must be having the same problems—and also aren't aware of the effects on their lives and on the lives of those around them.

Education is one of my specialties, and I do not understand why this information didn't become public knowledge long ago. I have access to a large library, but I can't find anything about beginning or mild hearing loss and its effects. Let's hope this book begins a trend until, as Alec says, this information becomes household knowledge, and the mysteries and miseries of hearing loss begin to disappear.

Alec has achieved what he set out to do. *Hearing Loss Help* is loaded with interesting information and practical suggestions—great stuff for anyone who has a hearing loss or who wants to help someone who does.

Good luck as *you* enjoy this book—just as I did.

> George Mulder, Ph.D.
> Counseling Psychologist
> Formerly Director of Counseling
>   and Testing at
> California Polytechnic State Univ.

TABLE OF CONTENTS

PREFACE

The background for this book began more than sixty years ago.

I look back on a lifetime of hearing with one ear only. I remember as a child how frustrated I was with being "different" from my brothers and sisters. I recall an almost constant effort to attract attention, to prove I was somebody. And a feeling of never quite "making it," or an emptiness when I did. I didn't know what was wrong.

Today, I do: No one could *depend* upon me to hear since I heard normally on one side and poorly on the other. And my first reaction to voices was a look of uncertainty as I tried to locate the speaker. I *was* different. Only recently have I become aware of how deeply hearing loss has affected my life.

When my good ear began to weaken, my communication problems got worse. I bought a hearing aid. It helped, but I still had troubles. I couldn't find anyone or any literature to answer my questions, "Why am I so frustrated? What can I do to make things better?"

To learn the **secrets,** I bought a hearing aid business —and got more frustration. Most of those with mild losses wouldn't even come in. Many of those who did refused the only help I had to give: hearing aids. Terrible. In a business selling only one product, amplification, with so many needy and so few takers. Real frustration.

But slowly, very slowly, I learned to focus first on *people* and *education.* And, I began to feel successful once more.

People want to know what's wrong and *practical ways to help themselves.* But, instead of telling them, we race on, becoming ever-more dependent on ever-better technology, and ignoring the most effective remedy for mild losses—education.

The entire subject of hearing loss is a mystery to most today—and it needn't be. Perhaps this book will begin a trend toward changing all that. It *does* focus on people and education.

P.S. In the three years since I wrote the first edition of this book, my hearing has gotten markedly worse. I now believe one of the most helpful things others can do for me is to let me know when they are about to speak so I can get "ready to listen."

When I'm not ready, I miss the first word or two ... and the rest is often meaningless.

But when others let me know they are going to speak, I nearly always understand quite well.

So now I ask them to *begin* by getting my attention.

INTRODUCTION: IS THIS BOOK FOR YOU?

First, this book is intended for those millions of "important others" who suffer right along with the hearing-impaired and long for *some way to help*.

Next, for those millions who have mild hearing loss, who aren't aware or don't understand what's happening to them and don't want to become locked in a life of loneliness and frustration.

I'll write just as if we were talking and I'll try to answer all *your* questions about hearing loss. Big words and complicated phrases or sentences will be scarce. Positive statements will be used since qualifying each to fit all situations would be far too cumbersome. This does not mean they are true in your life—you are the best judge of that.

Choose, just as in a cafeteria. Examine each idea or suggestion and picture it in your mind, your life. Accept it only if it seems right for you. And regardless of how it's written, this book will be of value to you only to the extent it makes sense to you *and* you are moved to act.

————

So here, reader, are the things I'd like to have known about hearing loss many years ago.

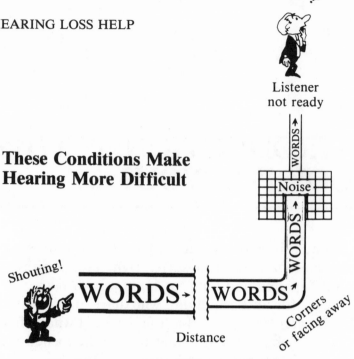

These Conditions Make Hearing More Difficult

Shouting!

WORDS→ ←WORDS

Distance

Corners or facing away

To improve listening conditions:

- **Don't shout**—it usually does **not** help.
- Instead, move **closer,** where it's **quieter,** where you can **face** each other.
- But even more important, begin with unimportant words so the listener is **focused** and **ready to listen.**

First, Get Attention...

This is one of the *most important* things you can do to help a hearing-impaired person hear and understand you.

To *get attention:*
- *call* his or her name and
- *wait* until he or she looks up
- *before* beginning your message.

These drawings are so important, they will be repeated whenever appropriate throughout this book. And each time they appear, their meaning will become more clear.

CHAPTER 1

HERE'S HELP FOR HEARING LOSS

If you are an "important other" in the life of a hearing-impaired person, *you* can make things better simply by learning to speak so you *are* understood. "Special speech" is something you can do on your own, and you can start any time. (Complete details in Chapter 13.)

Do you have a beginning mild hearing loss? Here, for the first time, is a practical approach which does not expect *you* to make all the changes.

And, for both of you, this book describes an effective program for reversing the ill effects of hearing loss:

1. Gather information:
   - get thorough *medical* and *hearing* evaluations to learn about your loss in particular.
   - read first twelve chapters of this book for general information.
2. Important others learn special speech.
3. You work *together* to improve listening conditions (including assistive devices).

These three steps pave the way for the success of the fourth:

4. Hearing aids.

In close relationships, *each* person suffers when one has a hearing loss. This book shows, step-by-step, how to overcome most hearing loss problems.

The focus is on *mild* or beginning hearing losses since there are many times more of them. But every suggestion helps those with *severe* losses as well.

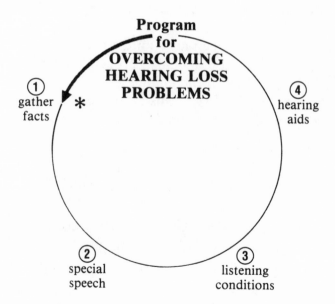

Program for OVERCOMING HEARING LOSS PROBLEMS

① gather facts ✱

④ hearing aids

② special speech

③ listening conditions

CHAPTER 2

MILD HEARING LOSS IS A MASSIVE PROBLEM TODAY

How Big?

The House Ear Institute now estimates 1 in 10 Americans are hearing impaired. More people are affected by hearing problems than all other major diseases combined. Obviously, there must be *many* millions more with unrecognized beginning or mild hearing losses.

> And each one's hearing loss affects at least one other person—altogether a huge and rapidly growing cause of unhappiness and misery in our society.

The Causes

The most common cause of hearing problems is a combination of the amount and kinds of noise you've experienced in your lifetime, and the accumulation of damage over time.

As we get older, this accumulation becomes noticeable in a gradual way. If you've been exposed to moderately loud noise through employment, hobbies, or environment, potential problems may show up sooner and be more severe.

Most hearing loss is the result of conditions over which we've had little control.

Examples:
- Noisy work places: Welding, stamping metal working, power saws, blowers, and so on. (Industry is gradually beginning to recognize this problem and take measures to protect their workers.)
- Living or working along busy streets with heavy traffic.
- Airport vicinities. It's estimated that at least half the general population near Los Angeles and London's Heathrow airports have hearing losses.

More hearing loss is one of the prices we pay for living longer in an ever-busier and noiser world.

Present Efforts Aren't Enough

Consider these figures from industry sources:

Twelve million hearing-impaired people (75% of 16 million) who could benefit from amplification (hearing aids) aren't getting it.

Approximately 1¼ million aids are sold annually. But far fewer people are actually helped since that figure includes the many who buy two aids or replacements, and some are bought and not used.

After ten years of intensive effort to promote the use of hearing aids, we may now just barely be helping people at a rate equal to the new cases being recognized. But 12 million (or more) still remain, year after year, without significant help.

Whatever the actual figures, surely it's obvious the present approach isn't meeting the challenge. But why?

Hearing aids *are* very good today,
and they often work miracles
—when accepted.

But when listening habits have been mostly lost and habits of silence and loneliness are well-formed, of course hearing aids *alone* aren't likely to reverse those habits.

The problem isn't with the hearing aids, it's with the "when accepted." Acceptance will continue to be a problem as long as we expect hearing aids to work in environments unprepared for them.

Fine aids alone aren't enough. The
"scene needs to be set" in order for
them to succeed, just as fine cars need
good roads. Education can provide such
environments.

Nationwide Education Needed

People want the "mystery" taken out of this whole subject, and when the mystery disappears, much of the present stigma will also.

People want to know all about hearing loss:

- How hearing loss affects their lives
  and relationships.
- How to recognize early warning signs
  and prevent these changes.

- How to create an environment where hearing-impaired people *can* hear.
- How to successfully encourage the use of hearing aids.

And when this knowledge gets to be a household remedy, much of the unhappiness now caused by hearing losses will disappear.

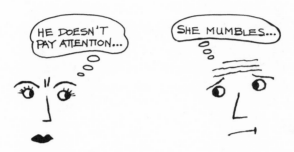

CHAPTER 3

HARRY AND EMILY— AND HEARING LOSS

Harry: "She mumbles; I hear men fine. Besides, I hear all I need to."

Emily: "He doesn't pay attention. I talk the way I always did. He just doesn't care."

His beginning mild hearing loss had been getting worse for years and now their marriage was threatened.

First, he began missing words in noisy places or at a distance. No problem, but he "did use *huh* and *what* more."

Next, he started misunderstanding at his weekly luncheon meetings and others looked at him "funny." Not bad, "just easier not to go."

He made mistakes on the phone, so he didn't answer unless necessary. But he "could get along without it."

The TV was either too loud for her or too quiet for him. Oh well, "TV's no good anyway."

He tried hearing aids . . . but "didn't like all that noise."

And so on, slowly withdrawing, slowly changing.

His reactions to his problems seemed natural and necessary to him. But when not hearing became habit, he was like a different person.

Emily was devastated. She enjoyed going out, the phone, the TV—she just liked to talk. And now he didn't.

Harry and Emily couldn't find information or help, so they waited . . . and suffered.

Their communication had changed, till now simple complaints were often blaming, hurtful, fault-finding accusations . . .

———

Now imagine this same situation existing in millions of homes today. Not a happy thought, but probably quite true.

CHAPTER 4

MEDICAL
AND HEARING
EVALUATIONS

When you do decide to get checked out for hearing aids, very often you'll go first to a hearing aid dispenser —either an audiologist who dispenses hearing aids or a hearing specialist (more on that later in this chapter).

The dispenser will ask questions, examine your ears, etc.—looking for anything unusual.

If the dispenser sees wax buildup, infection or anything abnormal, you'll be referred to a medical doctor. If this happens in your case, by all means have it done. Very rarely tumors grow inside the ear (unchecked, they can be fatal). Diseases, such as muscular dystrophy or diabetes, and metabolic disorders such as high cholesterol levels, can cause hearing loss. The first clues to these diseases often come from hearing examinations.

So, if your dispenser says you should see a medical doctor, by all means do so.

Chances are you'll feel relieved afterwards. Worry about our ailments is usually more destructive to us than the ailment itself.

"After all, our worst misfortunes never happen, and most miseries lie in anticipation."

(Balzac)

You'll be looking for answers to such questions as:

- Is the loss due to earwax or infection?
- What kind of loss?
- How bad?
- What about an operation?
- Is it permanent?

Licensed Physicians Who Specialize in Diseases of the Ear:

The prefix "oto-" means ear:

Otologist: a medical doctor who specializes in the ear.

Otolaryngologist: ear and throat.

Otorhinolaryngologist: ear, nose and throat, or "ENT" doctors.

How We Hear

Study the illustration on the following page: Sounds collect in the outer ear and vibrate the eardrum. In the *middle* ear, the three smallest bones in our bodies amplify and transmit these vibrations to the fluid-filled cochlea (part of the *inner* ear). There, hair cells convert the vibrations to electrical impulses. The auditory nerve

THE EAR

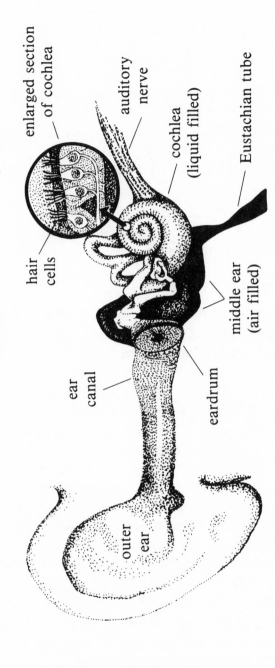

enlarged section of cochlea

hair cells

auditory nerve

cochlea (liquid filled)

Eustachian tube

ear canal

eardrum

middle ear (air filled)

outer ear

Sound (air waves) gathered by the outer ear vibrate the **eardrum.** Tiny bones in the **middle ear** transfer these vibrations to the **cochlea,** causing fluid waves inside. These waves bend the **hair cells,** generating electrical impulses which are carried to the brain by the **auditory nerve.**

carries these impulses to the brain—where they must be translated into meaningful sounds.

In any system this complicated, there are endless opportunities for trouble. Any problem in any part which slows or obstructs this process prevents normal hearing.

Hearing examinations show the kind of hearing loss and how bad it is. It may not be possible to tell you what caused your hearing loss.

Kinds of Hearing Loss

Here are some of the terms you may hear:

Conductive hearing loss.
> Sound isn't conducted properly from the outer or middle ear to the inner ear. Causes: obstruction in outer ear, punctured eardrum, infection.

> **Otosclerosis** is a type of conductive hearing loss. It's usually a hereditary loss in which the tiny bones of the middle ear no longer transmit sound properly from the eardrum to the inner ear. (Injuries such as car accidents may break these bones with a similar result.) Surgery often produces remarkable results with this type of loss. This is delicate surgery which is done under a microscope.

Sensory-neural losses.
> The inner ear is unable to properly transmit sounds to the brain. Causes:

severe German measles or mumps, high
fever, certain medicines, excessive noise.

Presbycusis is a hereditary type of sensory-
neural hearing loss that comes with aging. (This is where the phrase "normal
hearing for your age" originates.) The
hair cells inside the inner ear (especially
those for high-frequency hearing) wither
with age and no longer pick up sounds
properly. This kind of loss is permanent
since hair cells don't grow back. The
ability to hear high-frequency sounds
deteriorates nearly all our lives. Ex-
tremely high-pitched sounds we hear as
babies are often no longer heard by age
twenty. Usually both ears weaken
together. More men than women have
this type of loss and it's usually more
severe for men. Sensitivity to loud
sounds is common.

Permanent loss can also be caused by any disease or
condition which restricts blood flow to the inner ear,
such as stroke, injury, and so on. Certain antibiotics,
some diuretics for some people, even large doses of
aspirin can harm hearing.

Profound Hearing Losses

Severe losses are recognized as handicaps and great
efforts are being made to overcome their effects.

Examples: TDD and TTY devices (one typewriter-like device can "talk" to another similar machine over the phone). Many TV programs are now (CC) close captioned, so they can be read simultaneously on the television screen. Phones and doorbells can flash lights instead of ringing. Vibrators under the bed can be triggered by alarm clocks. And so on.

Cochlear implants are the focus of a great deal of research effort today. Sounds are converted to electrical currents which vary according to frequencies. By means of electrodes, these currents stimulate the inner ear to produce what the listener perceives as sound. Much of this work has been and is being done by the House Ear Institute in Los Angeles. The results are very promising for those with little or no hearing. However, the sound quality produced is *not yet* suitable for *mild* or moderate losses.

Audiologists and Hearing Specialists

These professionals are trained to identify and measure hearing loss. They choose and fit hearing aids, and measure the results in various ways.

In the past, these hearing aid evaluations were done by trying various different models. Today, fewer aids need be tried because most are adjustable for particular needs.

Both audiologists and hearing specialists have details about available help, financial or otherwise.

Hearing Aid Dispensers or Specialists

A license is now required in most states. In order to obtain such a license, a person combines study with training under a licensed person and then must pass a rigid examination.

These people were the **pioneers** in developing ways to deliver hearing aids to the public. They discovered practical ways to make up for equipment shortcomings, to overcome deeply imbedded customer resistance. They developed the sales necessary to finance today's remarkable hearing aids.

Audiologists

Audiology, or the branch of science dealing with hearing, is a graduate-level program that requires a minimum of a Masters Degree (M.A. or M.S.) (usually six years at the college level), and specializes in hearing examination and evaluation. Audiologists have at their command a wide variety of technology and knowledge that can help them pinpoint the particular causes of a client's problems and determine the proper treatment steps, including the critical skills needed to recognize those rare cases when medical or surgical help may be necessary.

Audiologists also spend considerable time learning the many important processes of rehabilitation and client counseling necessary for better hearing.

Successful hearing aid fittings result from:
1. The customer's need and willingness.
2. The dispenser's skill:
   - in testing.
   - in making comfortable, effective ear molds.
   - in choosing the most appropriate hearing aids.
   - and, probably most important, skill in helping the customers make the necessary adjustments so they can get the most from their hearing aids.

That last one is a real art. Each customer is different and a different approach is needed.

For more on this, see Chapter 19, page 123.

CHAPTER 5

GOOD HEARING HEALTH CARE

CAUTION

Get immediate medical attention for earache, drainage or sudden changes in your hearing. The sooner you do so, the less likely you will have severe or permanent loss.

External Ear Care

If you suspect you may have even a mild hearing loss, have it checked. Then you'll know.

Have your ears checked for wax buildup or any sign of abnormality at least once a year. Some people's ears produce enough wax to interfere with hearing in six months, others never. Earwax is bitter and sticky to discourage insects and other foreign bodies from entering the ear.

Do not use ear drops, cotton swabs, bobby pins or toothpicks to clean your ears. If wiping with tissue as far as you can reach isn't enough, get medical attention.

Anything small and long enough to reach the eardrum can puncture it. (Some eardrums are very fragile.)

Polluted water is a common source of ear infection.

Avoid poorly treated swimming pools and areas in the ocean or lakes where partially treated sewage is discharged (quite common in many areas today).

Eustachian Tubes and Earaches

These connections between our middle ears and throat serve to equalize the pressure on both sides of our eardrums.

When we are young, these pressures equalize rapidly and almost constantly. As we get older, these tubes become less active. Stuffiness from colds or hay fever also can block them.

When eustachian tubes are blocked, unequal pressures develop, causing earaches. The pain is usually worst in *planes* descending for landing or when driving down a mountainside. Outside pressure builds up and eardrums are forced inward. Many hearing-impaired people experience poorer hearing for various lengths of time after flying or long auto trips. This may be an effect of inactive eustachian tubes.

Check with your doctor before trying either of the following remedies:

Some people close their mouth and nose, and blow *gently* till pressure is equalized. (Be careful. This can blow germs into sinuses and middle ears.) Others get relief by taking decongestant tablets or using nose drops well before changes in altitude or after long trips when ears feel "stuffy." (Nose drops can quickly become habit and then do more harm than good. Use them only for short periods except on doctor's orders.)

Noise Pollution

Too much noise injures the hair cells inside the inner ear, causing permanent damage.

We are usually careful about loud noises, but continual moderate noises often do far more damage. Like most things which have no immediate effects, we don't pay much attention until too late—and then we pay the price. (This is how I weakened the hearing in my good ear—too much shotgun for too many years.)

Each step on the hearing audiogram (shown in Chapter 6) is heard as 3 times louder than the one before. Example: 90 decibels is heard as 3 times louder than 80 db. Some ears are more sensitive than others and can be damaged at lower levels but, on average, continual exposure over 80 db or any noises louder than 140 db can cause permanent hearing loss and/or tinnitus (see last section in this chapter).

OSHA (Occupational Safety and Health Administration) regulations say workers exposed to more than 85 db for 8 hours *must* have hearing protection.

Harmful Noises Outside the Workplace

Again, these are the most dangerous simply because we ignore them until too late. Harmful noises are *everywhere* in our lives.

If you already have a hearing loss, you may think you are immune. You aren't—overdoses *can* harm your remaining hearing.

Common Harmful Noises:

- Loud music. Those who want to "feel" music can certainly do so

today—with 150-watt speakers.
- Music through earphones can really blast.
- Power tools with piercing whines: chainsaws, circular saws, planers, grinders, etc.
- Motors: motorcycles, speed boats, snowmobiles, lawn mowers.
- Electronic arcade games.
- Ring signals on some cordless phones.

There is no OSHA to protect you in your private life—it's up to you.

Protective Devices

There are many kinds available today; the problem is finding the right kind for you. They must be comfortable or you won't wear them. Check first with audiologists or hearing aid dispensers. The next place is a busy gun shop (look under *Guns* in the Yellow Pages).
Types:

- Custom-fit earplugs are made to fit your ears only (usually by an audiologist or hearing aid dispenser). One kind has a valve which allows soft sounds such as voices or speech to pass through but closes for loud sounds.
- Disposable or reusable ear plugs, either separate or connected by cords or headbands. These are designed to

fit most ears just as they come from
the package.

- Ear muffs of all kinds. The pads
  which seal out sounds must be soft
  and spongy or they won't be effective.

Ear plugs must fit in order to shut out sounds and
clean to avoid infection. Most types give about 30 db
protection. Sometimes both plugs and muffs are needed
when shooting heavy firearms.

Tinnitus (Noises Inside the Ears)

Tinnitus means hissing, ringing, buzzing or clicking
noises inside the head. Loud and continuous tinnitus is a
terrible affliction—no rest, no escape. Its effects are
much like those of chronic pain: a feeling that *no one*
else really understands how bad it is. Feelings of frustration and anger, fear and stress follow.

Tinnitus is a symptom of injury or disease and very
often the cause can't be found. Some people are both-
ered more than others. For many, it's a problem only
when trying to sleep.

Because tinnitus can be a symptom of a serious
medical condition, treatment begins with thorough
medical and hearing evaluations.

Quite often tinnitus and hearing loss occur together. Sometimes *hearing aids* give relief from tinnitus.

Much has been done with tinnitus *maskers*. First,
tests are done to define tinnitus frequencies. Then an
appropriate masker is chosen. Some get help, others
think this is just one more noise they don't need.

Hearing aids and maskers are for waking hours.

Many things have been tried to help with sleep. Some people get relief from "white" noise produced by FM radios set between stations, or from tape recordings of waves, rain, and so on.

Much experimental work is now being done with *drug therapy,* chemical balancing, and electro-stimulation. The results are promising for the future.

In the meantime, there is one approach which does help those willing to try: *behavior modification.* This is a fancy name for learning to change the focus of our thoughts away from feeling sorry for ourselves to active interest in other things. It works. Perhaps we can't change our problems, but we *can* change our reactions to them.

If you can't find a tinnitus workshop, find one of those for pain therapy. They work and *are* available in most communities today.

Since there is often no satisfactory remedy for tinnitus, we should take all possible measures to prevent it or prevent making it worse.

We do know loud noises and some drugs (such as quinine or large doses of aspirin) cause ringing in our ears. When we're young, these noises usually disappear. As we age, such noises may become permanent.

———

Good ear care means using common sense *and* getting medical care when you need it.

CHAPTER 6

PHYSICAL EFFECTS OF HEARING LOSS

We hear someone talking. If we understand, we respond. When we don't, we say they aren't speaking clearly or loud enough. We don't think about the many things which must happen in order for us to understand words.

The Nature of Sound

Light waves, radio waves and X-rays are magnetic waves which can travel in a vacuum. In contrast, sounds are mechanical waves which travel through a medium such as air or water. Sounds are only a small part of the many mechanical waves around us: earthquakes, weather changes, ocean waves, and so on.

Sounds create tiny alternating high and low pressures as they pass through air. Each high pushes and each low pulls, causing our eardrums to vibrate.

There are many sounds we don't hear. And speech sounds are only part of those we do hear. The higher frequencies (up to 40,000 with some hi-fi speakers) are not heard, but improve sound quality by producing harmonics, etc.

Just as light is composed of spectrum colors, sound is made up of a range of frequencies. *Frequency* means the number of cycles per second (cps). One push and one pull together equals a cycle.

See the illustration on the next page. The page following that illustration shows an audiogram, a diagram which pictures hearing and hearing loss.

Hearing Tests

Sounds of one frequency at a time (puretones) are presented to each ear through earphones. The decibel loudness (volume) where these sounds begin to be heard determines the puretone hearing threshold or *hearing level* for that frequency.

Words and puretones are also used to determine the *discomfort* level, at which sounds become uncomfortably loud (but not painfully loud).

The *bone* hearing level is determined by presenting puretones more directly to the inner ear through a vibrator on the bone behind the ear (bypassing the middle ear). Marked differences between hearing through the air (earphones) and the bone are called *air-bone gaps.* They indicate *conductive* hearing losses.

Next, standard word lists are presented through earphones. A series of one kind is used to find the level where understanding *begins.* A series of another type of words presented at a comfortable level measures *how well* words are understood, or *discrimination* (usually stated as a percent).

Normal Hearing

"Normal hearing" abilities vary widely. The zero level on the audiogram is an average of the hearing tests of many thousands of people thought to have normal hearing.

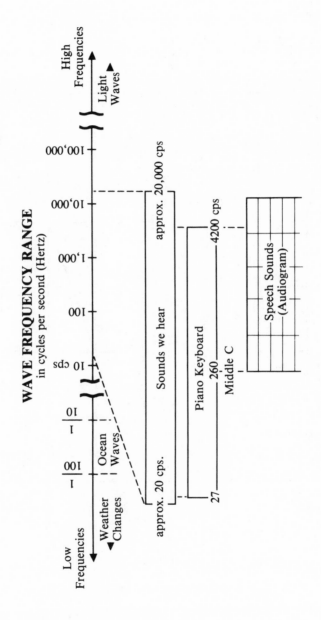

WAVE FREQUENCY RANGE
in cycles per second (Hertz)

High Frequencies

Light Waves

100,000

10,000

1,000

100

10 cps

10
1

100
1

Low Frequencies

Weather Changes

Ocean Waves

approx. 20,000 cps

Sounds we hear

4200 cps

Piano Keyboard

260
Middle C

27

approx. 20 cps.

Speech Sounds
(Audiogram)

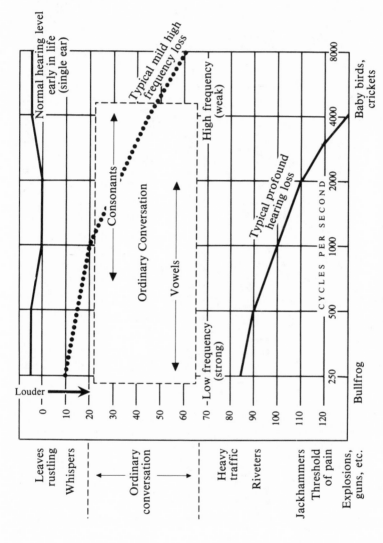

AUDIOGRAM: A picture of hearing and loudness

42

Normal Conversation

"Normal" speech also varies widely both in *loudness* and *frequency*. Some *word* sounds are strong and others weak:

> Vowels are *strong* low-frequency sounds which travel across distances well, turn corners readily and penetrate background noise more easily.

> In contrast, *consonants* are weaker high-frequency sounds. They fade quickly with distance, do not turn corners easily and tend to disappear in noise. (And there are *four* times as many consonants as vowels.)

At a loudness level where vowels are heard clearly, the soft consonants such as "s," "sh," "th," or "f" may not be heard at all. Others such as "p" or "t" may sound alike and be confused.

In addition, there are *strong* voices and *weak* voices.

"Are they easily understood?" is one of the first considerations in hiring newscasters. They must have *strong* voices. Voice strength comes from the use of lower frequencies and projection.

Projection means the air used to speak comes mostly from the diaphragm. It's natural for some people, others must be trained. High-frequency voices originating in the throat and upper lungs are *weak* and wispy in comparison.

> Habits which interfere with understanding:

Talking through teeth with mouth nearly closed.

Talking with hand over mouth.

Talking while chewing gum or eating.

Talking when it's noisy.

And there's more: Women's and children's voices are, *on average,* higher frequency and so, like consonants, more difficult to hear.

An example of the worst possible listening situation: A person with a weak high-frequency voice trying to speak around a corner, head in the cupboard, the water running and the radio on.

All of this applies to people with normal hearing. Now let's see how it is for those with hearing problems.

Hearing Losses

Hearing-impaired people live in a world which expects them to hear normally. They don't . . . And the conditions which make hearing difficult for people with normal hearing make hearing many times more difficult for those with hearing problems.

Mild losses are by far the most common type today. They are also by far the most troublesome because so few really understand what's wrong or how to help.

Look again at the audiogram at the beginning of this chapter. The dotted line shows a typical mild or beginning hearing loss. Mild losses have one outstanding characteristic: Strong sounds are heard normally and weak sounds are not. (This is why the term "percentage of loss" isn't practical for describing these losses.)

Now you can begin to see a more complete picture of hearing losses:

> Hearing loss is usually *greatest* at those frequencies where sounds and voices are *weakest*.

As people lose their ability to hear high-frequency sounds, they gradually compensate, often without awareness, by paying more attention to body language. Lip movements in particular are watched closely in effort to "read" the soft sounds (lip-reading, or more properly, *speech-reading)*.

The hearing-impaired combine what they see with what they hear, trying to form words and make sense. Then they guess, just as we all do.

———

For those of you with normal hearing, this has been all words and theory so far. Now for some experiments to give you the actual feeling of hearing loss.

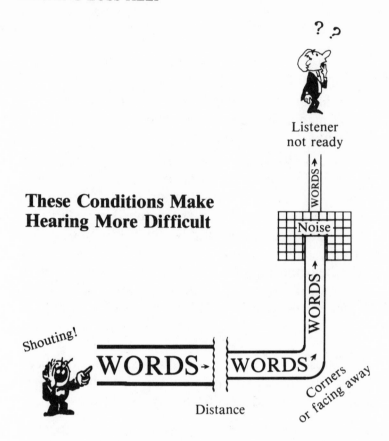

**These Conditions Make
Hearing More Difficult**

To improve listening conditions:

- **Don't shout**—it usually does **not** help.
- Instead, move **closer,** where it's **quieter,**
  where you can **face** each other.
- But even more important, begin with unimportant
  words so the listener is **focused** and **ready to listen.**

CHAPTER 7

HOW YOU CAN EXPERIENCE HEARING LOSS

If you have normal hearing, here's how you can create artificial conditions to help you understand the problems experienced by hearing-impaired people.

First, study the drawing on the opposite page. Whether you are an important other or hearing-impaired, you need to have this picture vividly fixed in your mind.

Distance

Even people with normal hearing begin having trouble with some voices and sounds at ten to twelve feet. Adjust a radio *only* loud enough to hear the *key* words and then move back three or four steps. Focus on what is being said and try to understand.

Stay with it till you begin feeling the uncertainty, the impatience, the *frustration*. How long before you want to turn it off and do something else? What if it were a person instead and you must answer? Could you respond intelligently?

Now focus on the *different sounds* and *different voices*. Which are more difficult to understand? Vowels or consonants? Male or female voices?

Noise Interference

Water is one of the worst interference noises. With the radio as above, turn on a water faucet or flush the toilet. The voices seem to fade into these "rushing" noises. Water makes a "white" noise which blocks out or masks nearly all speech sounds. *Wind* noise has much the same effect.

Other troublesome noises:

- Fans
- Microwave ovens
- Crackling paper such as when reading a newspaper
- Radios, TV's, hi-fi's
- Heavy traffic

Around Corners or Facing Away

Again with the radio just loud enough to understand at about ten feet. Without going farther away, move around a corner. The voices will fade markedly.

Now face away. The voices will be even more faint.

Listener Not Ready

Now think about a time and place (perhaps high school) when you were lost in a pleasant daydream and someone started talking to you. It took time to refocus and listen. Daydreams are places to think, to consider, to let the mind wander. With no critics except ourselves.

This is where hearing-impaired people retreat when others put them down simply because they didn't hear, when sounds are painfully loud too long. They go to escape, to rest.

They aren't *ready* to listen and will miss the beginning of anything said to them.

Lip Reading

We all do it.

Watch a TV newscast with the volume set where you can barely understand, close your eyes. You'll begin missing some key words. Repeat till you realize very clearly how much you depend on lip movements to help you understand.

So, if you talk to someone when turned away, it will be more difficult to understand you because your lips can't be seen *and* your voice will be weaker.

Loud Sounds

We all remember sounds so loud and painful we wanted to cover our ears and run. We each have different tolerances for continuing loud sounds. Hi-fi music at a pleasing level for some can drive others away. If you live with someone who has a hearing loss and turns the TV too loud, you know all about loud sounds.

Hearing-impaired people often lose much of their tolerance for loudness. The range between being able to hear speech and what is painfully loud may be quite narrow. Too much loudness too long makes us nervous or angry.

The next time you are exposed to a large dose of "loudness," think about the hearing-impaired who often face this problem daily.

Hearing With One Ear

Still listening to the radio at the same distance, hold

one ear tightly shut and slowly turn around. Notice how the radio sounds loudest when your open ear is toward it, and how much harder it is to understand when your closed ear is toward it. This is how it is hearing with only one ear.

Loss of Direction

When ears are unequal, hearing-impaired people lose their ability to sense where sounds originate. They often appear bewildered until they have located the sound source.

With one ear closed, close your eyes and stand still. Have someone move the radio around you, stopping now and then. Unless it's loud, you probably won't be able to point toward it.

———

Hearing-impaired people face such frustrations all of their waking hours, every day. The effects of these frustrations on their lives and the lives of those close to them are the subject of the next chapter.

CHAPTER 8

PSYCHOLOGICAL EFFECTS OF HEARING LOSS

Here are some of the many complex mental and emotional effects of hearing loss:

Uncertainty

Hearing-impaired people are balanced on the edge, between too loud and too soft, between hearing and not hearing—very often unsure about what's being said.

They are nearly always uncertain about what others think. We expect them to understand plain English. When they don't, we are puzzled, we frown—and leave to talk to someone who does. Losing half the ability to understand normal speech is much like losing the use of one arm, yet we help one and put down the other.

Quite naturally, hearing-impaired people stop exposing themselves to situations where continual stress and putdowns occur. *Withdrawal* begins.

They become more quiet—after all, it's their wrong responses which get them into trouble. At home, they are even quieter. Continually straining to hear is tiring and surely they shouldn't have to try so hard there . . . so "important others" in their lives feel neglected.

Worry

When we have problems, we worry: Will the rest of our lives be like this? No, "This too shall pass."

Worrying is nearly always a waste of time and strength, and does nothing but spoil our todays.

Repeating that quotation: "After all, our worst misfortunes never happen, and most miseries lie in anticipation." (Balzac)

Frustration

Now would be a good time to stop and look again at that short Chapter Three about Harry and Emily . . .

Harry was frustrated at his business lunches. The others didn't understand his problems and there wasn't any comfortable and effective way to tell them. He felt unfairly treated. He *withdrew*.

Emily was frustrated because he had changed and now she felt neglected.

They were both frustrated because they couldn't find information, couldn't get help. They felt helpless, lonely. Their frustrations built up until they began lashing out at each other.

Anger

Harry was angry with himself for getting older, being "weak." Angry at others for not really understanding his problems. Angry about hearing aids. Angry. He had begun looking for negative reactions and, of course, he found them—everywhere. More withdrawal. (For more about anger, see Chapter 12—Relationships.)

Emily had her own troubles. She too was getting

older, wrinkles appearing, children gone, menopause, a general feeling of worthlessness. And now, this hearing business! Harry wouldn't admit his loss, wouldn't do anything but wait. He was angry more often, his voice loud and unpleasant, and then *she* became angry.

Meanwhile, they waited . . . his not hearing was becoming a habit . . . their problems multiplied.

Stress

We recognize aches and pains as signals we are overdoing physically.

In contrast, we don't recognize the early symptoms of mental stress such as headache or indigestion. We simply take pills and go on. So mental stress often builds up into serious problems: mental depression, high blood pressure, heart disease, and so on.

Large problems such as death happen and there is little we can do but wait for the healing of time. We *can* do a great deal about the continuing small, nagging irritations, frustrations and worries which accumulate to become big problems.

Anger and worrying are mostly negative stress reactions and do nothing but damage. Yet, we continue to waste time and emotional energy on them day after day.

Withdrawal and the common habits which go with not hearing are usually negative reactions to the stress of not being able to hear normally.

Positive Stress Reactions

Some authorities say we worry most about our health, our looks, forgetting, losing things, having too much to do. There *are* positive reactions which do help.

Our health:

- We can't stop the natural aging process and worrying only hastens it.
- We can change our habits, eat better, exercise sensibly, keep busy.

Our looks:

- Worrying only adds more wrinkles.
- We can be clean, neat—and pleasant.

Forgetting or losing things:

- We can be patient and wait for the forgotten to flash across our minds, the lost to be found (yes, sometimes in the strangest places).

Too much to do:

- It's best if we *never* get *all* our work done. We need goals, something to anticipate, to keep us occupied.

Hearing loss must be approached the same way. We need to stop thinking about how bad it is and start searching for ways to help hearing-impaired people hear again and important others feel important again.

Most hearing losses worsen slowly, but their psychological effects feed on themselves and become bad habits far more rapidly.

Waiting is the very worst thing we can do. But before we take any action, we must be able to recognize mild hearing losses.

CHAPTER 9

EARLY WARNING SIGNS

Hearing loss comes without warning and can have drastic results before we realize what's happening. We can't prevent existing hearing loss but we can prevent or minimize many of the problems it causes if we recognize it early.

The process of changing behavior and forming poor listening habits begins when hearing loss begins. There are many signs.

Simple signs:

- Using "huh" and "what" more.
- Asking to repeat more often.
- Radio or TV too loud.

More complex signs:

- Avoiding groups.
- Avoiding strangers.
- Less TV watching.
- Less use of phones.
- Less small talk.
- More use of eyes, always watching.
- More silence.
- More withdrawal.

- More misunderstandings and arguments.
- More guessing, and more often wrong.
- More daydreaming or being "gone."
- More trouble with unexpected or rapid speech.
- Complaints about the way people talk nowadays.
- Punchlines often missed.
- Jerking head around to locate speaker.
- Startled looks.
- Perplexed looks.
- Impatience with interruptions.
- And the list goes on and on.

Regardless of how long the list, *behavior changes,* such as withdrawal and silence, probably mean hearing loss and that it's time to begin changing the things we can change.

CHAPTER 10

OUR NEEDS CONTINUALLY CHANGE

Needs are what motivates us to make our lives better: our desires, our wants, our longings. The "carrot on a stick" that leads us on. But before we can do anything about our needs, we must decide exactly what they are.

Abraham Maslow—On Needs

About mid-century, Abraham H. Maslow, an American psychologist, pioneered new concepts about human needs. It was an already widely recognized fact that we have instinctive basic needs for food and drink, security and affection.

Maslow went further. He contended that, *after* our basic needs are met, further instinctive needs appear. He called them *growth* or *being* needs or self-actualization.

Maslow saw our needs in a pyramid formation. The following page shows a more detailed version.

Maslow believed most of our needs at each lower level must be met before we are ready to begin satisfying our needs at the next higher level.

Dr. Thomas Gordon, another psychologist, in his book *Leadership Effectiveness Training* (see next

Unlimited—
Beauty, Goodness
Justice, Order, Wholeness
Approval Needs
(involving others)
Social Needs
(involving others)
Safety and Security Needs
Food, Drink and Warmth Needs

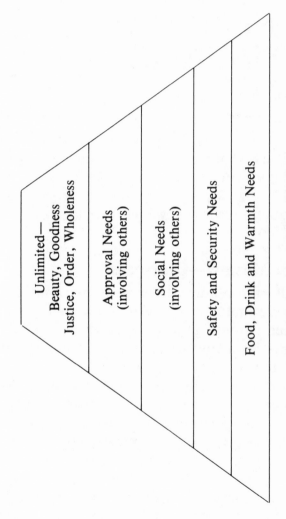

Maslow-type Pyramid of Needs

chapter) explains the process this way:

> "A primitive man who is hungry will be highly motivated to stalk a wild animal to obtain food, even risking his life (ignoring safety and security needs).
>
> "After killing the animal and eating what he needs and now motivated to satisfy his security needs, he may cure the remaining meat and store it for future consumption (safety and security needs).
>
> "When plenty is stored away, he then might think of asking friends to come over and share his food (needs for acceptance and social interaction).
>
> "When those needs are met, he may decide to experiment with a new and more flavorful way of preparing his food (needs for achievement, self-esteem).
>
> "Finally, if those needs are reasonably satisfied he might decide to paint pictures of the animals he has killed on the walls of his cave (need for self-actualization)."

More About Needs

As babies, we focus almost entirely on our own needs. As we get older we appear to become more outgoing as we are involved with others—marriage, children, churches, and so on.

But inwardly, we still focus most often on our own basic needs. Evidence: Our thoughts usually start within ourselves. "I wonder why . . . " "I wish . . . " "I think . . . " We argue and fight to defend *ourselves* and those important to *us*—and not often for our enemies.

We need approval by others and by ourselves in order to feel worthwhile, strong and ready to move on to better things. Those in the helping professions burn out unless they have their approval needs met by someone whose approval they value. Often this is another professional who "heals" them simply by listening and saying, "Hey, you're okay." Self-approval follows and strength to continue comes.

Many of us falter somewhere on the social or approval levels, simply because we don't communicate well. It's important to realize we have more than just basic needs. We need to feel good about ourselves. And, after that is accomplished, the top level remains: an *unlimited* area still to be explored.

We have a constant need for new goals, for moving from one set of goals to higher ones. As soon as we can look down from one mountain top, we begin looking for another to climb.

Most of us started pretty far down on that pyramid and now we've moved up. Our children, of course, want to start at the level they experienced when last living with us—and we often help them. So they start higher on the pyramid with fewer needs unmet, fewer opportunities to feel successful. And we wonder why they have such a time.

Different People—Different Needs

Heredity, training, teaching and life experience combine, making us all different. In addition, there are basic differences between men's and women's needs which are especially important to the hearing-impaired and important others.

Most of the people interested in this book will be from the generation born soon after W.W.I. These remarks are intended for them since discussions about sex differences are now no longer the style. Again, these are general statements to be applied to individuals only as they see fit (still the cafeteria approach).

First, men and women are physically different and one rejoices in that—how boring otherwise. On average, women's voices are softer just as their skin is softer (also nice). But softer voices are harder to hear. Men, on average, are more likely to have a hearing loss than women and their losses are usually more severe.

If the sexes are physically different, it's reasonable to assume they have differences in their thinking, their approach to solving problems.

Some psychologists describe men as more "linear" and women more "circular." Linear personalities start a project and drive toward completion, pushing things aside until done. Circular personalities manage many things at once, maintaining and making do.

For example, consider how a woman gets supper. She answers the phone as she stirs the gravy or as the cake bakes. She holds the baby as the toddler shrieks, "What that, Mommy," pointing to the blaring TV. And dinner is on time. *Patience.*

Now man. He puts the baby in the crib, the others in the living room, the phone off the hook and *then* cooks. "Let's get things organized here." *Impatience.*

Men also react differently to hearing loss, often to the detriment of themselves and others: they get impatient and do something. More than likely it's withdrawing to where they can get by and then fortifying this position. "I hear all I want to hear," "Don't bother me," and so on.

Women usually enjoy more touching than men. And more talking. Men want to be saying (or hearing) something they see as worthwhile. Most men want more silence and hearing loss intensifies this wish.

Retirement Needs

Both men and women have basic needs to be recognized as worthwhile. And many are not.

The woman: The children leave, a big empty house. Once so many important things to do, and suddenly so few. Menopause. Looks change. Everything changes. And now this man home all the time. He sits and watches and points out her inefficiencies—after all these years? "Am I nothing?" *Approval needs not met.*

The man: He retires. Big changes. Needs something to do. Here's this inefficient woman—ah, there's the first project and she doesn't like it at all. . . . Go fishing. Very exciting when there wasn't enough time, now flat when there is. What to do? No work, no play—no good? *Approval needs not met.*

Boredom

Retired and bored? Bored people don't endure.

They stop. They stagnate. No exercise, no interests—no hope.

Your enemy is not your ill health, your hearing loss, your mate. It's *boredom,* caused by a change in lifestyle from being active and useful to inactive and unuseful—and accepting this as fate.

Start making changes. Do *something.* Get busy. The daily routine of middle years no longer supports you and you must make *new* habits. There are always new projects to finish, new skills to acquire, new people to meet.

We Must Change Continually

"If we don't change directions, we'll
end up where we are now headed."
—Chinese proverb

Modern life teaches us to resist change. "Don't gamble, don't take chances, don't . . . " This is the *right* way and so on.

But we must change or life passes us by. Either way, we all continually go down that river of life. And if we row too long too many times upstream, fighting life, trying to stay young, we tire or our health breaks—and we drift right on downstream.

Tomorrow will be different. We will be one day older, one day less. Everything and everyone around us will be one day different. Will we change with it?

Change Thinking First

Except for instincts, our thought controls our actions. The trick to changing our thoughts (or reactions or actions) is to substitute another. Simply trying to *stop* is a prescription for failure.

Example: Change unpleasant thoughts to pleasant ones—a small project, a future fishing trip, reading and so on.

Make Small Changes One At A Time

Changes in what we think, what we do, how we relate to others. But take it easy. Trying to make too many big changes at one time is another prescription for failure.

As we focus on mountain tops, we often become uneasy, perhaps frightened. We tell ourselves, "I'll never make it," "I can't," "No use starting." But we can climb this mountain just as we've climbed those before it—one step at a time: "I can take this step," "I can make it to that boulder, that corner, that . . . "

Small changes, one at a time, until success becomes *habit:* "I've got that one done." Satisfaction. "Now I'll do this one."

Change Your Reactions

Repeating an earlier statement: We can't change many things in our lives, but we can change our reaction to them.

Examples:

- Change worrying and frustrations to problem-solving, focusing on what you *can* do and what you enjoy.
- You used to have a grip that made strong men cringe and now you can't even get that little cap off the syrup

bottle? Stop thinking about getting old and losing your grip—just get the pliers.

- Headache? Stop thinking about how bad it hurts and get interested in something worthwhile which you enjoy.
- Indigestion? As stress builds, food tolerance often falls. Try an elimination diet.
- Hearing loss? Accept the loss and start working on ways around it. Example: not loud enough? Move closer.
- And so on.

————

This chapter has been almost entirely about *our* needs and how we can change to meet them. But what if you need another's help? You "communicate" your needs. That's in the next chapter.

COMMUNICATION HAZARDS

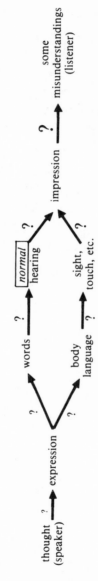

thought (speaker) ?→ expression

expression ?→ words

expression ?→ body language

words ?→ normal hearing

body language ?→ sight, touch, etc.

normal hearing ?→ impression

sight, touch, etc. ?→ impression

impression ?→ some misunderstandings (listener)

Communication is an uncertain business even with normal hearing—there are so many chances for error.

Good communication means understanding is essentially the same as the speaker intended.

CHAPTER 11

COMMUNICATING NEEDS

Hundreds of books have been written about communication and it's very difficult to condense so large a subject in one chapter.

Communication means transferring information. This information centers around our *thoughts* about our wishes, our needs. Whenever two or more people are together, communication of some kind occurs. The quality of our lives depends a great deal on how well we communicate.

Yet most of us know very little about it. We can talk and listen, can't we? But it's far more complicated than that. Example: silence can be very restful. It can also mean "I'm busy" or "I don't feel like talking" or "I don't feel like talking to you!"

Dr. Gordon on Communication

Dr. Thomas Gordon is one of the pioneering giants in the field of teaching better communication to parents, to teachers, to leaders.

Well over one million people in the United States and 16 foreign countries have attended his Effectiveness Training Courses.

His approach is simple, straight-forward and effective. Quoting with permission from his book *Leadership Effectiveness Training:* (New York: G.P. Putnam's Sons, 1977)

> "Effective communication with real understanding is much rarer than most people think because:
>
> • People don't always feel free to say what they really mean.
>
> • People are not always in touch with their real feelings.
>
> • Feelings are somewhat hard to put into words (it's hard to find the right code) . . .
>
> "As a rule, people don't get down to the real problem until after they have first ventilated a feeling or sent some opening message, such as:
>
> • I should have stayed in bed today.
>
> • Oh, forget it.
>
> • If it isn't one thing, it's another . . .
>
> "As everyone also knows, all people don't share their problems with others freely and openly. Sometimes, because we're not aware of what's bothering us, openly articulating our feelings can be difficult. Admitting to others that we are experiencing a problem may not be easy because we fear we'll be judged and evaluated negatively or subjected to irritation or anger . . .

"It is important to understand that one never *knows* exactly what another person is experiencing, because it is impossible to be inside the other person's skin. All you can do is *guess* what is going on inside another, relying on interpretation of the messages you hear, whether verbal or nonverbal . . .

"We can never be absolutely certain we have completely or accurately understood another person, so it is essential to test the accuracy of our listening and minimize the misunderstanding and distortion that occurs in most interpersonal communication . . .

"Real understanding of another person happens only when the receiver's (listener's) impression (the results of decoding) matches closely what the sender (speaker) intended in his or her expression . . . "

And later in his chapter on Turning Conflict Into Cooperation:

"Let's put our heads together and see if we can come up with some solution that would meet the *needs* of *both* of us . . . " [And that's the real purpose of communication.]

You will find complete details in any of his three books (available in most libraries): *Leader Effectiveness Training, Teacher Effectiveness Training,* or *Parent Ef-*

fectiveness Training.

For information on his seminars, call (619) 481-8121 or write:

Effectiveness Training, Inc.
531 Stevens Avenue
Solano Beach, CA 92075

You will be richly rewarded for every effort you make in learning to communicate better.

Verbal and Nonverbal Communication

Nonverbal (body) language is a combination of tone of voice, facial expression, position of hands, body posture. Understanding it is nearly always just guesswork. So, we need appropriate words to help us understand clearly.

Some experts say our communication is as much as 90% nonverbal and nonverbal is stronger. If we must make a choice and body language is apparent, we will very likely believe the body language regardless of what is said.

Examples: If someone says "I'm okay" and their body says not, we believe the body. When we meet someone who rubs us the wrong way, we usually don't even give them a chance to prove otherwise.

Others understand us most accurately when our words, tone of voice, facial expression, hand positions and posture all say the same thing.

Good Listening

The people we like best are those who really *listen* to us. There aren't many. True listening is hard work and very few of us can do it accurately more than a few words or sentences.

Good listening means fitting our verbal and nonverbal impressions together and then guessing fairly correctly just what the speaker intended.

Our most common fault—we simply *stop* listening.

We hear *trigger* words or phrases and stop listening to examine our reactions to what was said. Example: When a public speaker uses a word we don't know, we stop listening while we are thinking about its meaning in that context. We hear what interests us. In groups, we listen to certain voices. And individuals in a group listening to one speaker hear different things.

Or a trigger word or expression catches our attention and we stop listening as an answer flashes into our thoughts. Then we work on remembering and can hardly wait for the other to finish talking. And, of course, we are responding only to what was said before the trigger word.

We talk and talk—but we don't listen.

Good Communication

Good communication happens when the listener's *understanding* closely matches the speaker's *intention* and, as far as possible, the needs (or desires or wants) of *both* are satisfied.

Our communication (and lives) improve as we focus on eliminating the need for guesswork: We *speak clearly* so others needn't guess and we, as listeners, also don't guess. We make sure we *understand clearly* before we respond.

Expressing Ourselves

If what you say is important, treat it that way. Say it in a way so it has a good chance of producing the desired results.

- Consider what has happened before-hand. Ask yourself, "Is now the best time to talk about this?"

- Communication is usually good when we feel good. Incomplete messages are okay, jokes and teasing are appropriate then. But, when we are upset, angry or ill, it's very difficult to express ourselves without making matters worse. This is a time to be very careful. It's much better to say, "I don't feel well—could we talk about this another time?" than to say hurtful things we don't really mean.

- We are more aware of others' body language than our own, so we need to be aware of how we appear to the listener. If we want our message to get results, our verbal and nonverbal languages must agree.

- Don't expect others to read your mind. "They should know that" type of thinking leads directly to misunderstandings.

- Think about what you want to say. Plan. Commands, demands and threats work only as long as you can enforce them *and* others don't end the relationship. Common results: resentment, anger, rebellion—use only in emergencies. Rewards work only as long as satisfactory rewards are available *and* others can't reward themselves. Leads to dependency.

- Think about how to make your message effective. Have reasonable reasons, state them clearly and rely on the other's sense of fairness. This is the strongest appeal we can make. Leads to cooperation.

Listening to Others

It's easy to listen, right? Besides, we usually know what's going to be said and so on. Take another look. Listening is far more difficult than talking. For serious matters, you must:

- Consider what went before. When you don't feel good, your reactions may not be appropriate. Could it wait? If not, be very careful.

- Or, when the other person doesn't feel good. We must not react to the first statement when others are ill, upset or angry. It will very likely be inaccurate and may be entirely unrelated to the actual problem. When we react to these often-wrong first messages, arguments nearly always follow.

- Watch body language—theirs and yours. To listen well, you should be interested.

- Focus on what's behind what's being said, and *not* on your response. You can't do both. A proper answer requires a clear understanding of the speaker's meaning.

- Try to form a habit of not responding (except in emergencies) until you are sure you really understand. Slow down, study body language, inquire.

- *Then* make your best guess and *check* it out. Ask questions. "You say . . . " "You mean . . . " "You feel . . . " Get the full story before trying to respond.

Top sales people are successful because they listen well. They ask leading questions and listen until they determine what we want. *Then* it's usually easy. Mail-order ads succeed to the extent accurate guesses are made in advance about what people want.

Meeting Each Other's Needs

If our needs are stated clearly at the right time and listening is well done, meeting each other's needs is often automatic.

If not, focus on negotiating, compromising, cooperating (whatever you want to call it):

Instead of thinking how unreasonable the other person is, focus inside yourself. Is this something you can or should judge? *Does it really matter to you?* Is there a way to satisfy the other's needs without making problems for yourself? (There usually is—if we look.)

Communication Rules

1. Choose appropriate times, when you both feel good mentally and physically, when others are ready to listen.
2. Have something to say and say it clearly.
3. Don't stop listening till the speaker is finished.
4. Be willing to look for the common ground where the needs of both are met.
5. Practice—till habit takes over.

Communication and Hearing Loss

In today's society, we *expect* others to understand us, yet they often don't, even with normal hearing.

Those with hearing problems of course have more communication problems. Think about how much more often they must *guess*. As they lose their ability to hear words, they become even more sensitive to body language, creating more guesswork. Where guessing goes wrong too often, psychological changes begin. And these changes are likely to cause far greater problems than hearing loss itself.

People with hearing losses tell us, over and over,

what they need:

"If only people would talk plainer."

"I can't hear when she's around the corner or in the other room."

"I can't hear when the water's
running."

"I can't hear when the radio or TV are
playing."

Sometimes I'm a stubborn listener. When people
came to see me seeking help and made remarks such as
the above, I immediately set them straight: "They're
not mumbling—you just don't hear as well as you used
to." Right?

Wrong! I heard these pleas for many years before
finally "hearing" their real message:

"I need help—plainer talk and better
listening conditions."

Important others also have needs which are usually
unstated: to be understood, to be appreciated, to feel
worthwhile.

———

Good communication means successful
relationships.

CHAPTER 12

RELATIONSHIPS

Most relationship problems come from poor communication, *not* from thoughtlessness or selfishness. Nearly all of us are *willing* to help others *if* we understand that there are good reasons for doing so. This means we must *listen* to discover these reasons and others will help us—if we ask properly.

Relationships are partnerships and dissolving partnerships is a primary source of income for lawyers. We expect partners to *help* us meet our problems. Often we get new and greater problems instead. Relationships are difficult at best and require *constant care* in order to survive. In whatever form, this care means good communicating. First, the serious problems.

Anger

Anger is a secondary reaction which follows a more primary feeling such as: fear, pain, helplessness, frustration.

We hearing-impaired people are often angry. (I grew up full of anger. Others didn't seem to understand me or approve of what I did, and nothing I tried changed those feelings of helplessness and frustration.)

We, who have lived with anger a long time, are likely to fall into habits of dominance. We give orders and commands, not because they are right, but because we are *we*. And we enforce them with anger. These demonstrations hurt others and we don't feel very good for having steamrolled another. Sorting out the "peck order" is fine for chickens, but not very rewarding in close relationships.

When we are angry, our body language overwhelms our words. Our voices become harsh, we frown, tempers flare and all our problems are magnified. Immense amounts of time and energy are wasted. And we continue, time after time. Preventing all anger is, of course, impossible and not desirable. But most things we fight about aren't worth nearly all that time and effort. Most will be forgotten a month from now.

There are many theories about anger and how it should be handled. Some people promote anger expression as a way of managing others and getting ahead. Others say, "Use anger to make relationships more exciting and vital." Somewhat like using whips to improve sex?

Unreasonable anger is great—in relationships we don't want to preserve.

It's true: we shouldn't bottle up anger. If we do, it's likely to burst out all at once and make a mess. But, instead of looking for ways to express anger, how about looking for ways to remove the cause, such as feelings of helplessness, frustration or pain.

A wise man once told me, "Oh, we get angry all right—we just don't get angry at the same time." It took me just ten years to get the full impact of that statement: *don't respond to anger with anger.*

Anger heaped on anger starts fights—and wars. If you want to *lose* an argument, answer anger with more anger. It's like throwing gasoline on a fire.

The effects of the anger-habit are headache, upset stomach, diarrhea or constipation, high blood pressure and the like. Do we really want to spend all that time and effort on being angry?

If you want to *win* an argument, listen and listen and listen. The results will be truly rewarding.

Listening does many things. It calms others' anger. It gives time for our first angry response to fade. And we just might see a sensible way to meet the other's needs without causing us problems. The next time you are angry because of another's anger, *stop*. Forget that smart answer on the tip of your tongue and *listen*. Notice how quickly the tension begins to leave your body. Then practice until listening replaces anger and becomes habit in *your* life.

Meeting Each Other's Needs

When we're single, we are often frustrated and lonely, a captive of our freedom. When we form close relationships, we pay another price—some of the things we think we'd like.

Pleasant relationships exist somewhere in a compromise region, each of us getting our needs met most of the time. To find this region, we first must listen and learn each other's needs. We mustn't assume we know the other's wants and we mustn't expect them to know ours. (Jumping to conclusions is a poor way to get exercise.)

Keep in mind, our needs do change. As we get

older, we often want different things. Example: One may want to travel and the other to stay home, where the chairs fit and the toothpicks are handy. Instead of trying to force the issue and making both unhappy, why not go separate ways part of the time? Time together afterwards will be better for it.

We men are often real experts in this compromise business in our personal lives. We get so wrapped up in our own thoughts and projects we have little time for really listening, for really caring, for a hug or even five minutes of serious conversation on a topic of the other's choosing. We've been "in charge" so long we don't even think about compromise.

Talk and touch, listen, inquire, negotiate, give and take—these are the secrets for making relationships blossom.

Rewarding Relationships

Again: A happy couple we admire. We call them well-adjusted. Each seems to know what the other needs and acts accordingly, acceptably. Words are often only a small part of their communication. A few words, a look, a touch and they know. You can see it. They've spent a lot of time learning each other's likes and dis-likes, and they've learned how to fit these needs together into a rewarding relationship.

Tragic things happen. They pick up the pieces and go on—together.

They are experts at living—together.

Relationships and Hearing Loss

Hearing loss brings out a lot of anger in some people. And sometimes, the hearing loss itself makes voices seem louder and more unpleasant than is actually intended. So special efforts are needed to be sure communication is well done.

Consider that happy couple again. If he has a hearing loss, what then? Focusing on meeting needs, not blaming or finding fault, she has already discovered how to make him understand. (She wants to.) He has learned to listen more carefully. (He *wants* to hear *her.)*

They intend to keep right on communicating regardless of hearing difficulties.

Hearing loss can actually make relationships better if the end result is more touching, more thoughtfulness, more understanding.

———

Reviewing those four steps for overcoming hearing-loss problems:

1. Learn about hearing loss.
2. Special speech.
3. Better listening conditions.
4. Hearing aids.

We have now worked through hearing loss and its effects and we're ready to take action.

First and most important—special speech.

These Conditions Make Hearing More Difficult

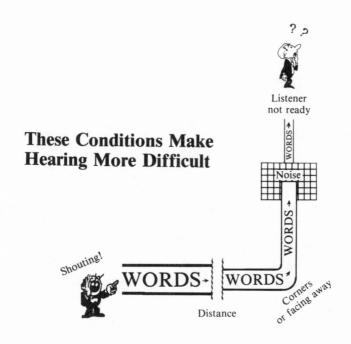

Listener not ready

Noise

WORDS

Shouting!

WORDS → WORDS

Distance

Corners or facing away

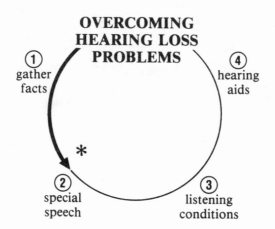

OVERCOMING HEARING LOSS PROBLEMS

① gather facts

④ hearing aids

*

② special speech

③ listening conditions

CHAPTER 13

SPECIAL SPEECH

Speaking so you can be understood is easily the most important thing you can do to improve your relationship with a hearing-impaired person.

Special speech will be *your* individual contribution to *your* relationship. You won't need money or permission or cooperation—only willingness and persistence. And you can start whenever you want. Like now.

Reviewing the problems faced by hearing-impaired people: not being ready to listen, weak sounds, weak voices and interfering noises. They are balanced on the edge of hearing, between too loud and too soft, between understanding and not understanding. When words are continually missed and body language misread, terrible things can happen. *Uncertainties* fill their lives.

They have a desperate need to *understand* their important others at the very least. And you will find many of your own frustrations disappearing as soon as *you* begin speaking so you are understood.

Again, keep in mind the most common reasons for not hearing (see drawing on opposite page).

Special Speech Rules:

1. Attract their attention.

2. Move *close* and face them.

3. Speak *slowly* and distinctly.

4. Wait or move closer when it's noisy.

You'll see results almost at once when you begin making these four simple changes in the way you speak.

Now let's examine each rule to see why they work so effectively:

1. Attract their attention. They must be ready to listen or key words at the beginning of messages will be missed and the rest meaningless. They need time to change thoughts and focus on you. Use other beginnings such as names, touching or unimportant words: Example: "Harry, about so-and-so" and *then* your message.

2. Move closer to make your voice louder and clearer. Face them so they can "see" the word sounds on your lips as you talk. Also, your voice fades rapidly around corners or when your back is turned.

3. Speak slowly and distinctly. *We* hear and *we* understand. The hearing-impaired do not. They must combine uncertain hearing, body language and guesses into words, and then into meaningful thoughts—often one step at a time, a slow business. When words come too rapidly or are slurred and weak, systems overload

and shut off much like electrical circuits, and listening stops.

4. Wait or move closer when it's noisy.
Even people with normal hearing
have trouble when it's noisy.

Other Points to Consider

Watch carefully as you speak. Stop whenever you
see signs of uncertainty—something has been missed.
Rephrasing may be necessary for the severely impaired,
but it often confuses those with mild losses. They don't
want another message to decipher, they just need to
know the missing key word or phrase (usually at the
beginning). Start again, watching to be sure you *are*
understood.

Don't shout. With mild loss, loudness alone usually
doesn't help, and often hurts. Worse, you may sound
angry.

Save important talk for appropriate times. Busy
people interrupted thoughtlessly usually aren't happy
listeners. And you may be training them to ignore you.
Ask yourself, "Is now the time to talk about this?" *A
caution:* talking to hearing-impaired drivers can be
dangerous—driving may be forgotten as they turn to
look for visual cues.

Be sure about important matters. Prevent costly
misunderstandings by discussing money, legal matters
and so on only when hearing conditions are ideal.

Be especially careful when either of you is ill or
upset. Discussions often turn quickly to anger in these
circumstances.

If your special speech doesn't seem to be working,

it is probably because your body language or your tone of voice conflicts with your words. When words and body language disagree, the hearing-impaired are likely to believe body language or may simply stop listening.

Practice, Practice, Practice

Keep a copy of these rules handy to review whenever needed. Experiment and practice until using them becomes habit. Be patient with yourself—you'll forget and they'll forget, but stay with it.

You want better listening to become a habit also, but again, be patient. You can't force listening—you must wait for it to happen. Try, observe reactions, and try again.

First, practice one-to-one in quiet. When that gets better, work on ways to manage in more noisy or busy places. Leading the way without smothering or over-protecting is quite a challenge—think before you act and try to avoid putdown situations.

Example: People with mild losses can usually understand one-to-one, asking questions when unsure. If you are present, doctors and others may talk to you since it's easier, and the hearing-impaired may be ignored. Discuss this and decide in advance.

Special Speech and More Severe Losses

Special speech helps with all hearing losses, not just mild ones. However, if you must talk to someone with more than a mild loss, you'll need to follow these rules even more carefully. In addition, it will help if you speak slowly and distinctly, and "project" your voice.

Projected voices are more forceful and have the

same effect as moving closer. You can learn projection on your own well enough for most hearing-impaired people. Practice in private so you don't feel uncomfortable. Start by saying "Gr-r-r-r" or "Br-r-r-r" as deeply as you can. Hold your throat and chest muscles tight and rigid, making the pressure for talking come all the way from your stomach. When you get it right, you'll *feel* your voice in your diaphragm as well as in your throat. Then practice doing this with other sounds until you can project your voice whenever there is a need.

If you have trouble, someone who teaches singing probably can help you. If you would like even more help, check with an audiologist.

———

Remember, the object of special speech is overcoming uncertainty. Continually look for better ways to eliminate guesswork in your relationship. Nothing else you can do will be as rewarding.

The harvest of happiness is most often
reaped by the hands of helpfulness.

—*This Way to Happiness*
by Gilbert Hay (New York:
Simon & Schuster, 1967)

COMMUNICATION HAZARDS

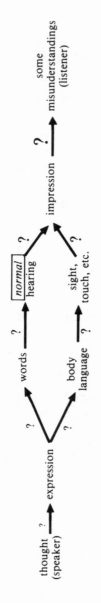

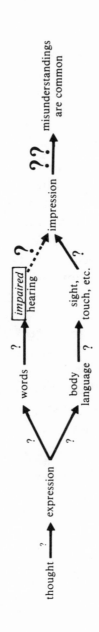

As hearing weakens, misunderstandings multiply.

Whenever you are uncertain, don't guess—say why (not ready, noise, etc.), and try again.

CHAPTER 14

HOW THE HEARING-IMPAIRED CAN HELP THEMSELVES

I am hearing-impaired—no eardrum in my left ear since age two, and now little high-frequency hearing in the right. I look back on a lifetime of uncertainty: about what I hear, what others mean, what they think. I have developed a whole batch of deeply ingrained not-hearing habits, from an often loud and harsh voice when excited or upset to a love of silence, a complacency with being alone.

And I wonder how different my life might have been with normal hearing. But might-have-beens don't cut any wood, they just make us sad.

From now on in this book, I'll be speaking as a hearing-impaired person and giving examples of how it was (and is) for me, and from my experience as a hearing aid dispenser.

What You Can Do

All right, you've had medical and hearing evaluations and you have a "permanent" hearing loss. First, face facts.

Once our listening systems start to get "warts," we're usually stuck with them, just as with the wrinkles on our faces. Hearing is one of our most complicated body functions. Restoring normal hearing is like restoring part of the brain—not yet possible. Without some miracle, we'll have to live with our hearing losses. How well we do that is up to us.

We can't change our hearing losses, but we can change our reactions.

Our Usual Reactions Often Fail

We often begin by denying our problem and then we defend our position with remarks such as these: "I hear okay," "I hear some people," "People don't talk as plain as they used to." We stall and wait—and form habits of not hearing, of silence, of withdrawal, not listening. These habits are very difficult to change and some of us end up leading a hermit-like existence—amongst people.

After a while we decide to try hearing aids. We've always had them in the back of our minds as a last resort—and now they don't help. It isn't that we *won't* wear them, it's more like we *can't*. Our habits have changed and aids seem to interfere more than they help.

We're really upset now. We wait more and our poor-listening habits become more fixed.

Well then, what reactions will help? Back to basics. Our problems are centered around uncertainties. First, work on those caused by poor communications, using better listening and better ways to ask for help.

Listen Better

When an important other in your life makes special efforts such as special speech to help you understand, the least you can do in *fairness* is stop and listen. Otherwise you'll be training them not to try.

Your biggest problem will be in not being ready to listen. When you are busy or your thoughts are far away, you need a signal to start listening. Stop and look up whenever you get that signal. Then make sure you understand. Ask questions to be sure—this is no place for thoughts such as, "If it's important, it'll be repeated." And be alert for the other's problems. We're so wrapped up in our own troubles that we often overlook theirs.

I've replaced one of my not-hearing habits with a better one: when my wife speaks, my mind shuts off and I focus on her. This took a lot of practice, but it happens almost automatically now and makes up for a *lot* of my other sins. The power of listening is so strong—if only we would remember to use it more often.

Asking For Help

We are handicapped and we need help. We must ask for it in ways which don't offend others. This sounds simple. It isn't.

First, we must tell them what's wrong. When someone with only one arm fumbles at a manual task, people want to help them. When we (with only half of normal hearing) fumble with words, people look at us as if we aren't quite right—because they don't know what's wrong. People know what to do when they see white canes, but when we say we don't hear well, they shout at us and then wonder why we frown in pain. And we withdraw even more.

Someday the general public will know exactly what we need when we say we don't hear. In the meantime, we do the best we can.

Hearing loss is not a disgrace; it's a communication problem and these problems are solved by better communications. *Defend* yourself. Say what's wrong. *Every* person whose relationship you value should know all about your hearing problems and what you need to understand. They won't unless you tell them and it's not *fair* if you force them to guess instead.

Being open about hearing loss is a real challenge. Start carefully with those close to you. Experiment until you find the ways most comfortable for you. Each time you succeed it will get easier. I've worked at it till now it's natural for me to say:

> "I have a hearing problem. Please don't
> shout—it hurts. I need to watch your
> mouth as you talk."

When others understand your problem, they will try to help you (or you'd better look for other friends). But they still don't know what you need in order to hear. *You* must know exactly what to tell them and how to say it. It helps to keep in mind how we hearing-impaired people understand speech:

- We must first stop thinking and get ready to listen.

- Then we try to locate and watch the speaker.

- We listen and watch, trying to fit together sounds, lip movements and body language.

- We try to form words, then phrases and finally thoughts.

- Sometime during this process, we must identify the subject matter or those thoughts will be meaningless.

- We guess (we want to keep this at a minimum—wrong guesses in wrong situations do harm to our self-esteem).

As you listen to others, think about these steps and learn to identify where understanding stops. Then whenever you don't understand, *you* will know why and you *can* explain to others. You'll find that you need to help people help you by continually reminding them *why* you didn't understand.

Messages That Work

People respond to requests for help *if* those requests don't offend *and* there is a good reason to do so. Tell them why—don't expect them to guess. Your frame of mind should be, "I want to hear what you have to say. In order to hear, I need . . . "

Those *non-blaming requests* for help do get cooperation. Dr. Gordon calls them "I-messages." Examples:

"*I* didn't understand."

"*I* missed the first word."

"That noise blocked out your voice."

In contrast, *blaming* requests usually produce anger. Dr. Gordon calls them "You-messages." Examples:

"*You*'re mumbling again."

"Why do *you* always talk around the corner?"

> *"You* keep saying I should get hearing
> aids."

And try to stop those "huhs" and "whats." Others often take them as criticism of the way they speak.

To make a believable and forceful message, your non-verbal language (posture, expression and tone of voice) must indicate you want to hear. Watch your tone of voice particularly when excited, upset or frustrated. Emotions mixed with hearing loss can make voices loud and unpleasant, having effects exactly opposite those wanted.

Watch *what* you say also. When one or both of you are ill or upset, the first remarks that pop into your heads are often poisonous. Stop, listen and think. Do you really mean that? Do you want to take the time and energy to deal with the consequences? Most important of all, will it have the desired results?

———

Better listening and better messages are two tools you can use to make your life better. Another way is to improve listening conditions.

CHAPTER 15

BETTER LISTENING CONDITIONS
• SITUATIONS

You are the expert on *your* life, so continually look for new ways to help yourself hear.

Remember, how you hear depends a great deal on two conditions: how close you are to the sounds you want to hear and how far away from interfering noises.

For instance, in your home: Arrange the seating so the person you want to hear most often is nearby on the side of your best hearing. Sit so you are closer to the TV and as far away as possible from kitchen and bathroom noises. Simple, but very effective.

Interfering Noises

Many noises are intermittent and you'll be able to hear between them (such as airplanes passing overhead). But you must both understand the need to stop and start over if necessary, whenever it's noisy. When the noise is continuous, try to move closer, or move your conversation to a quieter place.

If you work where it's noisy and you must hear, ask to be moved to a corner, along a wall or into another room. If you own the business or have clout, have a soundproof office built. You'll get a lot more work done and you won't be nearly as tired at the end of the day.

Now let's look at some special situations.

Children

Children have high-frequency voices and often duck their heads and lower their voices in shyness. But they *are* very willing to help us—all we need do is explain what we need and why.

And a hug or pat on the back makes up for a lot of not hearing (with adults also).

Small Groups

Small groups, such as family gatherings, can be very difficult for hearing-impaired people. Words come rapidly. You don't know who'll be talking next. Many will be turned so you can't see their faces. Others are waiting to jump in with a quick comment. It's often noisy. You feel lost, left out. Manage so you have a little special time with each one, explain your hearing problems, and let them know you care.

Try not to withdraw from groups you like. Make your problems clear so they understand you aren't anti-social. Since most of our language is nonverbal, you can still enjoy being there even if you don't hear all the words.

Places of Worship

Many now have public address systems. If so, you'll need to move around to find the best hearing. For me, the back row is usually the best. There is an audio speaker nearby and that person (who'd like to lead the choir but hasn't been appointed yet) won't be letting go right behind me.

Some places now have audio loops (see next chapter for details).

Again, even if you don't hear everything, you can enjoy just being there.

Crowds

In crowds, even people with normal hearing lean toward each other and shout. For you, it's babble, and there's little you can do except try to move your conversation to a less noisy place. If you'd like to talk with one or two, ask them to come to the edge of the crowd or go for coffee—or some place to get away from the noise.

Movies—Theaters—Plays

Actors, in trying to act naturally, raise and lower their voices and turn away. Often there's loud music in the background. All this makes it very difficult for many hearing-impaired people. If loud sounds aren't a problem for you, by all means go and enjoy the entertainment.

I've stopped going to most. The music and voices are of course aimed at the majority (who like it loud). It hurts me and there's no place to hide. So, I wait and watch it on TV. I can turn my remote listener up and down and understand most of it (see next chapter).

Restaurants

Try to sit in a corner or along a wall away from the kitchen or cash register noise. Experiment to find the best place for you.

When you find a location you like, ask for the table number so you can reserve it in the future. Try sitting next to your companion rather than across the table or booth. You will be surprised how much better you hear (and you might like it there).

The people who wait on you often have weak voices and look down at their order pads as they ask what you'd like. Study the menu beforehand and give complete orders in advance, from kind of salad dressing to cream or not in your coffee. Then there will be no need for questions or answers.

Understanding Professional People

You go to see your doctor. He speaks with his back turned as he looks down at your chart. You miss his comments and ask him to repeat. If someone with normal hearing (perhaps younger and more attractive) is there, he soon switches over and talks to them instead because it's easier and quicker. You begin to feel like a pet at a veterinarian.

I go alone. Professional people soon realize what I need in order to understand because I keep telling them when I don't hear *and* why. If they are too busy, I make another appointment to talk only—or find another doctor.

Or course, someday my hearing may get so bad I must have an interpreter, but not yet, thanks.

How to speak to the hearing-impaired will someday be taught in professional schools and receptionists will be taught the simple art of speaking directly into the phone, and so on. In the meantime, you are on your own.

Impossible Situations

There will be some situations where there is no satisfactory way to let strangers know you have a problem or how to help, and all you get is misery.

Examples: Stores which have young salespeople who like to *feel* the loud background music as well as hear it. You can't hear and they have trouble understanding you (they've already begun losing *their* hearing). Or a busy supermarket with people talking nearby, registers ringing, that background music again.

Avoid such places whenever possible. If you must go, do the best you can and then leave. (Store managers take note: do you want to continue discouraging or driving away up to 20% of *your* customers?)

Cautions

When important matters (money, legal, and such) come up, sit face-to-face where it's quiet and be *sure* you both understand.

Be careful when driving. Traffic and wind noises interfere and you may forget driving as you look for visual cues to help you understand. This is a place for the other to use forceful special speech. Encourage it and appreciate it. Inside cars is also a great place for an FM personal listener with a lapel microphone on the speaker (see next chapter).

———

Be inventive. In every situation, look for ways to get closer in order to hear and farther to avoid noise.

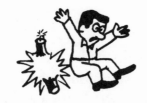

First, Get Attention...

This is one of the **most important** things you can do to help a hearing-impaired person hear and understand you.

> To *get attention:*
> - *call* his or her name and
> - *wait* until he or she looks up
> - *before* beginning your message.

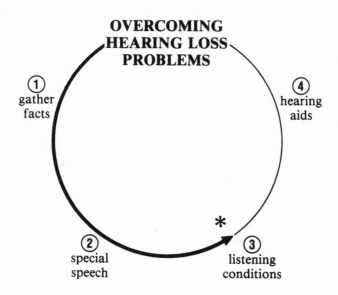

OVERCOMING HEARING LOSS PROBLEMS

① gather facts

④ hearing aids

② special speech

③ listening conditions

CHAPTER 16

BETTER LISTENING CONDITIONS
• ASSISTIVE DEVICES

Assistive device in this case means any device other than hearing aids for helping hearing-impaired people.

In the past, assistive devices have been promoted mostly for people with severe losses. Little has been said about how much nicer they make the lives of those with mild losses. Think seriously as you read these pages. There is a great potential here for making lives less frustrating and more pleasurable.

Assistive devices are nearly always better buys than hearing aids for all purposes or situations in which they do the job more effectively. Example: even when hearing aids are on and working, many people can't hear the ring of most phones from a distance. And what about at night when aids aren't worn? Hearing aids are simply not the best tool for listening on the telephone or to TV, and buying them for that purpose is often an expensive and disappointing mistake.

Some of these devices alert us, others help us hear better.

Alerting or Signalling Devices

These devices signal when phones or doorbells ring, to awake us, etc. They remove many of the uncertainties which go with hearing loss: "Did the phone ring?" "Was that the doorbell?" In fairness to relatives or neighbors, fix the phone so *they* aren't uncertain: "She doesn't answer—I wonder if she's all right?"

The most common signalling devices simply make sounds louder. For example, phone ringers can be placed in several parts of the house or outdoors. For the severely handicapped, other devices use flashing lights to signal phones or doorbells ringing. Alarm clocks can operate strong strobe lights or vibrators under pillows or mattresses.

Telephone Listening Devices

You need to be able to hear over the phone so you won't dread hearing it ring when you are the only one there to answer. And so you can maintain contact with your important others who do use the phone.

I must have a phone, but I often resent the thing. Whenever a salesperson stops taking my *cash* money to talk to a *prospective* customer, I'm reminded what a rude instrument it is. It intrudes. It demands. We're carefully programmed to run when it rings. Yet, it can be life-saving and today's life would be impossible without it.

The telephone will become even more important as computers become more common (they'll be talking to each other). So get comfortable with using it.

Here are some of the problems you face:

- Background noise.
- You don't know who's calling.
- You don't know what they'll talk about.

- They usually talk rapidly.
- They often don't talk into the mouthpiece.

Defend yourself. Your message goes like this: "I have hearing problems. Please help me by talking carefully directly into the mouthpiece." This is much better than having them wonder about your mental facilities.

Background noise will be less if you have your phone in a quiet part of the house. (If you use an extension cord, be careful about tripping over it. Such cords are a major cause of accidents in the home.)

If one of your ears is better than the other, learn to use the phone on that side. Practice in private so you'll have your writing hand free. If you wear a hearing aid in your best ear, you may do better by removing it. You need a tight seal against your ear to shut out noise and "squirt" the sounds directly into your ear. In noisy places, it may help to hold the other ear closed. (Be sure not to leave aids behind, especially in phone booths.)

Dr. Paul Hartman, San Diego, suggests covering the mouthpiece when listening to cut down on noise interference.

The simplest assistive devices make the voices louder. An amplifier phone is available from your phone company. This is usually more costly, since it's an on-going expense.

Some hearing aid dispensers and some phone shops have modestly priced amplifiers which fit *between* the handset and the body of the phone (see photo next page). Complete amplifying handsets are also available. Your phone must have the new modular handset connection in order to use either of these devices (see following page).

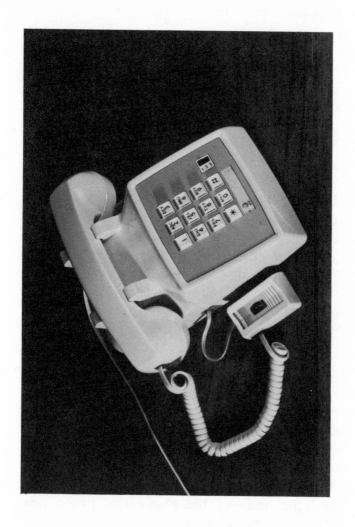

Amplifying Phone

One widely advertised amplifier has an elastic band which holds it against the earpiece. These work, but have two drawbacks: they usually must be removed before the phone will hang up and they use expensive batteries which go dead overnight when you forget to turn them off.

Hearing aids with T-coils pick up magnetic voice signals from *some* phones and you can adjust the loudness with the volume control on the aid. If this T-switch doesn't work on your phone, usually the phone company will exchange it for one that does (inquire about change-order charges). Or you can get a slip-on adapter which creates its own magnetic field. These adapters are great on vacations, business trips, and so on. But, you must have an aid with a T-switch.

Perhaps, someday in this age of miracles and miniaturization, someone will market a slip-on adapter which works on all phones with or without hearing aids, and has an automatic off switch.

Telephone Answering Machines

One of these is another device for helping hearing-impaired people. No matter how much we object to them, they are a fact of life today and people are beginning to accept their use. Ask pleasantly and people with important matters *will* leave messages.

These machines help by removing much of our surprise, our unreadiness to listen. You then can think about what you want to say and how to say it without the pressure of trying to do this while trying to understand.

Get one on a trial basis and see how it works for you.

Telephones and Tape Recorders

Many reasonably priced attachments are available for connecting your tape recorder to phones (again, ask for return privileges).

Ask for permission to record important messages so you can study them later. That way you can concentrate on what is being said and proper responses without having to make notes at the same time.

———

My phone equipment?
An amplifier on the home phone and a wife who amplifies for me away from home when it's noisy. Also, an answering machine and tape-recording equipment.

Television

If we want to keep our ability to process
sounds into words and complete
thoughts, we must practice continually.

When we stop both socializing *and* watching TV, our listening practice stops and we lose the habit. We say it's because the programs are "no good." Many of the programs are terrible today (particularly for our generation), but there are also many good ones. We need to find them, get interested and make listening part of our daily routine. Besides giving us listening practice, TV is a great device for overcoming boredom and loneliness.

One of the first steps in solving TV-listening problems is to sit as far as you can get from kitchen or bathroom noises. "But," you say, "I still can't hear or it's too loud for others." Right—the way it is. So *fix* it.

You need two things: the sound louder for you and a convenient way to adjust the volume for different voices and commercials. Remote control sets are very nice, but will *not* serve the same purpose. The sound *must* be louder for you than for others. Various devices work quite well. Some are connected to the set (wired), others are wireless.

Wired TV Listeners

For years, one simple type of wired device has been given away as promotions or sold for a few dollars. They have buttons on one end to go into the ear and clips on the other which connect to wires inside the set. There are problems: The sound quality is poor, there is no volume control, and they can be a shock hazard.

Cautions:

Any wired remote listener should be connected to the set through an appropriate isolation transformer to prevent the possibility of shock. The earphone outlets on most new sets are already transformer protected.

Wires on the floor are a great hazard in homes. Install wires under the carpet or around the wall—*or be careful.*

For the best understanding, you need sounds right on the edge of being too loud. You must have volume control so you can turn up for weak voices and down for loud commercials.

Earphones *with* volume controls connected to the earphone outlet will work fine. Problems: earphones are usually uncomfortable when worn over long periods. And using the earphone outlet shuts off the set so others can't hear.

Remote TV Listening Devices

Find a way to hear and understand TV comfortably. You will enjoy it more and others will appreciate your thoughtfulness. *And* it will help you save your hearing ability. I've heard this statement hundreds of times, "Oh, I don't need that." But *you do need it.* You'll understand why—when you try it.

For mild to moderate losses, the new *infrared listening systems* are a joy to use. With the new light weight earphones, the sound is released very near the eardrum and the high frequency sounds are much clearer.

For severe and profound losses, *FM listening systems* are almost a requirement. These systems can also be used in other situations wherever "loops" are available—classrooms, auditoriums, churches, etc. (see next section). Many of the personal listeners described in the next section work for TV also.

Group Listening Systems

The systems were developed for people with severe losses and are a great help. They could also help those with mild losses, but acceptance is of course even more of a problem than for hearing aids.

The Quota Club and the SHHH organization (see

108

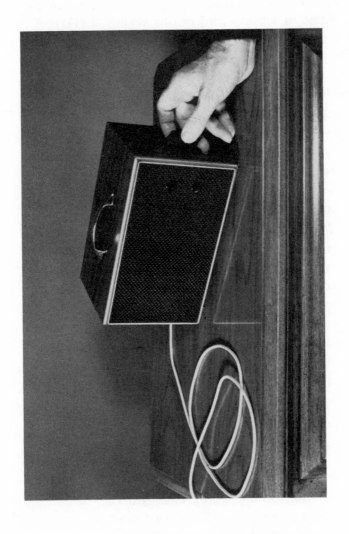

Remote Speaker (wired)

end of this chapter) actively support installations of these systems in schools and public rooms. SHHH also provides current information about where and what type of systems have been installed (they have extensive computer files).

These are the most common types:

- *Audio Loops:* Sounds are converted to magnetic forces and travel through wires under floors or around the walls. Hearing aids with telephone switches (T-coils) pick up these forces and change them back to sounds.

- *FM Systems:* Easy installation. Trans-mitters broadcast sound just as radio stations do. The listener uses a per-sonal receiver for making sounds available to the ear. The present trend seems to be toward this type, since in-stallation is easier and signals can be picked up for long distances.

- *AM Systems:* Same as FM except more static-prone.

- *Infrared Systems:* These are the new-est. Sounds are converted to infrared waves and back to sounds again by the listener's infrared receiver. Easy installation and static-free, but the range is limited and infrared waves won't pass through obstructions such as walls or around corners.

Other Personal Listening Devices

There is a wide need for appropriate personal listeners to help people with mild to moderate losses who are unable to use hearing aids, yet need to hear part time. (See the last section in Chapter 17.)

———

If you aren't confused with all of this by now, I am. Written words (and even pictures) are not the way to learn about devices this expensive. Except for wired TV listeners, almost all of these devices can be tried in *your* home. *Try* them first and don't buy something you can't use.

Tape Recorders

We mildly hearing-impaired people can get a lot of good from tape recorders. Not only for phones, but for seminars, in classrooms, meetings, etc.

Most teachers and seminars will let us tape record if we ask first. Reviewing these tapes later, as slowly and loudly as we need, gives more opportunities for reflection and reinforces learning.

Continually look for other ways to use a tape recorder in your life.

Buying Assistive Devices

Begin by getting the two most important (and lowest cost) items: a telephone amplifier and remote TV, speaker. After you've seen how helpful they are, think about others.

Most of the more expensive products are available for trial in your life and your home—there is no other way to be sure.

There is a great deal of confusion in this field today. Many companies are flocking into the market, yet no one seems to have a workable plan for distribution. As evidence: the January-February '85 issue of SHHH Journal lists *only* 12 centers offering substantial displays of assistive devices.

At any rate, you'll need *current* information about where these devices are available. One of the best sources is:

SHHH
Self Help for Hard of Hearing People Inc.
7800 Wisconsin Ave.
Bethesda, Maryland 20814

This is a rapidly growing organization with local chapters across the country. Dues are modest, the help extensive. Examples: A journal every other month, a list of available information filling both sides of a legal-sized sheet, effective lobbying efforts.

SHHH is intended for all hearing-impaired people, but of course those who don't admit they have losses also don't participate. This situation is slowly improving as hearing-loss problems become more widely recognized and understood.

Another source of information about assistive devices is *The Voice* (Paula Bartone, Editor, 712 Enchanted Harbor, Corpus Christi, Texas 78402, (512) 888-5747 Voice/TDD.)

Writing this chapter has been very frustrating and discouraging for me.

I've called many firms across the country. Some have answering machines promising return calls and nothing happens. Others have people answering who don't even know how to talk on the phone to be understood, and don't know their merchandise.

I called as a person with a mild loss. The standard response went like this: "Oh, these are for people with severe losses. What you need is a hearing aid." Sure, I need a hearing aid. But, first, I need appropriate assistive devices.

How long will they so completely ignore their largest market: me and the ten million others like me?

Enough.

Get the simplest and most important devices first. They can be gifts from others or simply gifts from yourself to yourself.

And each one will make your life a little easier, a little better.

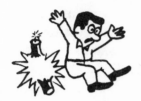

First, Get Attention...

This is one of the **most important** things you can do to help a hearing-impaired person hear and understand you.

To *get attention:*
- *call* his or her name and
- *wait* until he or she looks up
- *before* beginning your message.

CHAPTER 17

OUR ELDERS

Our Frustrations

As we watch our parents get older, we imagine how it will be for us and we become uneasy.

In sympathy and frustration, we look for something we *can* do for them. Aha! We'll get them hearing aids so they will hear as they did years ago (yes, trying to make them young again).

Some are quite willing. Some hate the very idea, but they may try just to please us. Think and study carefully before you begin this program. There are better things you can do first.

Hearing aids are usually not a problem for the elderly who have already learned the habits of using them. But for those first-timers, learning these new habits is often a terrible task. They have trouble with putting aids on, with keeping them working. Probably an even greater obstacle: they have grown comfortable with the habits of not hearing in their quiet world and they don't like "all that noise." Yet they do want to be part of things and they are caught. Don't add to their problems by being pushy.

Many times a son or daughter brought a parent to my office for hearing aids. I would try to be alone with the hearing-impaired long enough to discover their true wishes. And so often someone's dainty grandmother would say with tears in her eyes, "But I *don't want* a hearing aid!"

What You Can Do

First and most important: careful special speech, especially tone of voice and expression. Short periods of warm, meaningful conversation are far better than hours of lukewarm time. Work at it.

Next, assistive devices: Get telephone ringers or signalling devices so they know when you call, amplifiers to help them understand you. Get TV amplifiers so they can hear and enjoy the TV without bothering their neighbors (see Chapter 16).

After that, if they *want* to try hearing aids, help them.

Rest Homes

Rest homes are also places where we "see" our future (yet estimates say only one in twenty of us will ever be there). These places cause real problems for hearing-impaired people. Some statistics say 80% of patients have hearing losses. Many who are thought to have mental problems simply can't hear.

Most hearing aid dispensers quickly learn to avoid rest homes because they are nearly always ineffective there. It's difficult for middle-aged people to accept and use aids, and it's almost impossible for aged non-users to learn how. One can put on aids and they work fine as long as someone helps. Too many things can and do go wrong: They forget how to put them on, to turn on or adjust the volume. Batteries go dead. Aids get put through the laundry with the bedclothes or become wrapped in a facial tissue and thrown away. Complete frustration for the user, their relatives and the hearing aid dispenser.

There's another complication. Some patients groan or moan continually. Severely hearing-impaired patients are used as "buffers" to separate these groaners from those with more normal hearing. Fair? Practical, at least. When one puts hearing help on these buffers, of course, they don't like it. As my father said, "I *don't want* to hear others hurting."

As a result, almost nothing is now being done for these hearing-impaired people. Surely, they should at least be provided with some way to hear better for the times when they *do want* to hear.

Needed: A New Type of Assistive Device

Some kind of device is needed allowing workers and relatives the ability to talk with severely impaired people without straining, so that the hearing-impaired can hear whenever they wish.

I've spent eight years and thousands of dollars trying to develop and promote such a device. For various reasons, no company seems interested. And now *I'm* getting old.

Someday, someone will market a device along these lines:

- Stethoscope-type earpiece to fit everyone.
- Large controls for stiff fingers.

- On / off switch with indicator light.
- User volume-control with large numbers and long rotation. (Needs a lock for those unable to manage otherwise.)
- User tone control such as on hi-fi systems.
- Master volume control for different losses.
- Automatic gain control for loud sounds.
- Portable.
- Reasonably priced (well under $100).
- Needs to be marketed as an assistive device only to avoid restrictions.

———

In the meantime, do what you can. Use your best special speech. In particular, get close. Above all, make your voice and expression pleasant and let your good nonverbal language speak for you.

CHAPTER 18

ACCEPTING HEARING AIDS

So now you are thinking about hearing aids? If you are starting here in this book, consider going back, reading it from the beginning. Here's what you need to know *first* to insure success:

- Why you don't hear.
- How to tell others.
- Help from important others.
- Better listening conditions (including assistive devices).

Be sure you have in mind the *four most important obstacles* to hearing (drawing repeated again on the following page).

You may have tried aids before and didn't like them. Try again now as outlined above. Your hearing has probably gotten worse, hearing aids better, and your approach will be more appropriate.

Hearing aids are a bonus for mild losses: the finishing touch in your program for solving your hearing loss problems.

We Resist Hearing Aids

We have an *unreasonable* resistance to hearing aids

These Conditions Make Hearing More Difficult

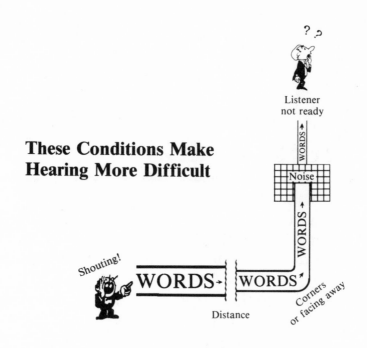

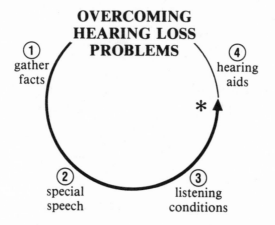

much like our resistance to seat belts. (Yet we are twice as likely to survive a serious accident when wearing them.)

We justify this resistance by making comments like these:

"I hear all I want to hear." (Really?)

"I'll get aids when I need to." (Waiting too long seems to go with hearing loss.)

"Too much money for that little thing." (Not if it works.)

"My neighbor says . . . " (Forget the rumors and find out for yourself.)

Our Unrealistic Expectations

The general public thinks first about hearing aids for hearing losses. Important others pressure us to get them. Advertisers say aids *are* the answer. We soon believe they are and they become our fall-back position.

So we wait, and then when we do try, we often don't get what we expected (loudness alone doesn't do it). Now we really are upset and we have a new excuse, "Hearing aids are no good—I tried them."

What We Can Expect

Here is an honest and fair statement:

For mild losses, hearing aids used properly are very effective in quiet places and are well worthwhile for that reason alone. The results won't be as good when it's noisy, but the newer aids are

beginning to overcome a great deal of
the "noise" problem.

Requirements for Accepting Hearing Aids

- Good listening conditions.
- Help of important others.
- Willingness on your part.
- Time, effort, and patience.
- Aids must be physically comfortable,
  or they won't be worn.
- Sounds they produce must be comfort-
  able as well.

CHAPTER 19

BUYING HEARING AIDS

Hearing aids *are* very good today. Your job will be to get those which help *you* hear better.

Choosing a Hearing Aid Dispenser

Try to find a dispenser who gets results. Ask your doctor, your neighbors, your friends. Not what is the best kind of aid, but who is the best dispenser.

Next, study the dispenser's advertising. If it sounds too good to be true, it probably is. Knowing what I know now, the most negative thing for me would be signs of high pressure (such tactics and competence may not come together).

Gimmicks, words and phrases such as these could indicate high pressure:

- "Free." Is anything really free today?

- "Electronic testing" or "Electronic hearing aids." Just another way of saying electrical.

- "For nerve losses." Most of us have nerve losses and that's when hearing aids perform their best.

- "Separates speech from noise."
Speech is noise, but many aids actually
can filter out much of the most offen-
sive background sounds and also block
feedback.

Try to meet the dispenser. You'll be working
together during the trial period. Will you be able to
cooperate? Watch and listen as you sit in the waiting
room, or wait outside and quiz departing customers.
What is the dispenser's attitude? Are problems blamed
on customers or does the dispenser *listen* and try to
overcome those problems? Does the dispenser provide
and firmly believe in *good* trial periods? And so on.

Usual Terms

Today, it's common for dispensers to require a
deposit, perhaps half the total price of the aids and to
retain part of this for testing, etc., if you decide not to
keep them.

Whatever the terms, be sure you understand and
get them in writing along with receipts. In the excite-
ment of "being able to hear again" and, with so many
subjects discussed, you may not remember everything.
Keep an ongoing record of what was done, on which
date.

Buying hearing aids is one of the few areas today
where you *must* be helped or you needn't pay. If you
buy a car, you've bought it, "lemon" or not. If you buy
hearing aids properly, you won't be stuck with any
"lemons."

Know Your Legal Rights

Laws vary from state to state, far too much to cover here. Most states have written or implied regulations about warranties. In California, the law says you have 30 days to decide whether or not the hearing aids are doing what you need. If not, explain the difficulty to the dispenser and it must be remedied or your money refunded—but you must act within 30 days. If you do return the aids and are unable to get a refund at that time, be sure to get a dated receipt.

Good records, timeliness and persistence together usually win in disputes about hearing aids.

Aids now must have the date of manufacture stamped on them. The dates are difficult to find on some brands. Ask the dispenser to show you. There is usually a lag at year-end and some aids sold early in the year will be dated the previous year. This is nothing to worry about.

Used Aids

Used aids may appear to be bargains, but be very careful. Even if you buy for half price, they may not last half as long. Worse, the hearing results may not be even half as good as they could be.

Hearing Aid Prices

Don't be overly concerned with prices. If aids work, they are a bargain. If not, don't buy them. Hearing aids are costly, but the price has not increased nearly as much as medical costs, groceries, etc.

Severely impaired people must have hearing aids

and assistive devices, usually regardless of cost. And a great deal of financial and other help is available to them. This is not true for those with mild losses. Yet we *can* somehow find money for the things we *really* want.

Aids which end up unused in a dresser drawer are a complete waste of money. Look for good hearing instead of bargains. After the trial period, decide: do the aids make your life better? If so, by all means buy them.

Being Good to Ourselves

As we get older, the things the doctors don't restrict —we can't do any more. Or, we don't want to. I remember when I was thirty and a tiger at fishing and hunting the Colorado high country. I thought how terrible it was that Dad didn't want to go along. Now that I'm in my sixties, I don't care much about going either. As we get older, there are fewer and fewer things we can do for ourselves that really make our lives better. Hearing aids can do that.

———

Maybe we should stop trying to save it *all* for tomorrow or for our children, and spend some for living better today.

Typical
Hearing Loss Problems

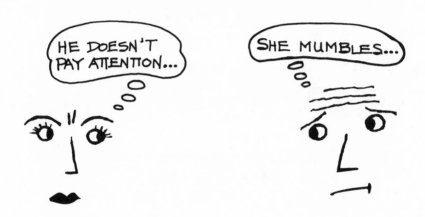

Does this sound familiar?

**If so, perhaps it's time you
did something about it.**

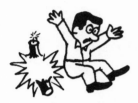

First, Get Attention...

This is one of the **most important** things you can do to help a hearing-impaired person hear and understand you.

To *get attention:*
- *call* his or her name and
- *wait* until he or she looks up
- *before* beginning your message.

CHAPTER **20**

TYPES AND BRANDS OF HEARING AIDS

Hearing aids are somewhat like a public address system. Sounds are picked up by a microphone, made louder and sent through a speaker to the eardrum. Hearing aids are much smaller, and the smaller they are, the more difficult and expensive it is to get good sound quality.

Hearing aids not only make sounds louder, but they must make certain sounds louder than others in a pattern which fits individual losses. Hearing aids should also be capable of protecting against loud sounds for persons sensitive to them.

One Aid or Two?

We were given two ears for good reasons. There is little doubt that two aids (binaural) are better than one for almost everyone who can benefit from amplification.

Sounds will be clearer and stronger. Two aids produce a stereo effect much more like normal hearing so you can sense direction again. Regaining your sense of direction reduces feelings of confusion and helps you locate the speaker and begin picking up visual cues sooner. You'll act and feel more alert.

Wearing two aids is particularly important if you are working, meeting the public, etc.

Balancing the volume controls may be a problem at the beginning. Learning takes time and practice, but soon becomes automatic.

Many people who have used a single aid for years and get a second, then say, "I wish I'd done this long ago." If you wear one aid only, *try* another which matches yours, or two new ones, and then decide.

With a single aid, you must resist the temptation of turning it too high to make up for both ears. Otherwise, you won't find a comfortable setting so you can wear the aid continuously. (See the section on volume control adjustment in Chapter 21.)

Types of Hearing Aids

Since this book first appeared, aids which fit entirely within the ear have become very common. They account for well over two-thirds of the aids fit today.

Because of new ways for controlling feedback, they may be effective for more severe losses.

All-in-Ear (AIE) aids have the microphone, amplifier, and speaker all within a case made to fit the inside contours of each individual's ears (see photo on page 131).

When these aids were first marketed, durability was a problem. Now better materials and technology eliminate most of these troubles.

Depending upon how your ear is shaped, removal may be a problem. Ask about "removal" notches or knobs. Wind blowing across the microphone openings makes some aids roar. Remedy: wind screens. Some aids have screens to keep ear wax, dead skin, etc., from

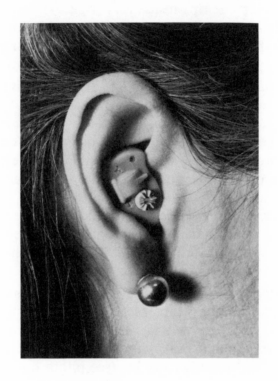

All-in-Ear Hearing Aid

plugging up the tips inside ears. Ask.

Many dispensers include extra molds for use with behind-the-ear loaners if your aids need modifying or repair.

Canal aids are the least visible of any. They fit in a small shaped space at the beginning of ear canals (see photo on page 133).

The sound quality of these aids can be quite good since the bowl of the ears is open to help collect sounds, and the tip is closer to the eardrum for better high frequency hearing.

Discomfort may be a problem for some people during long periods of wearing. Canal aids are of course easier to drop or lose. The cost is usually higher and the durability less than with other types.

Low-profile aids use the same full-sized cases as regular AIE aids, but have an inset face plate so the microphone, battery cover and volume control are recessed. They are less apparent, wind noise is reduced and the ear bowl helps gather sounds (see photo on page 134).

Behind-the-Ear (BTE) aids hang behind the ears, with connectors and tubing going over the ears to carry sound to the earmolds (see photo on page 135).

For years these were the aids of choice and are still preferred by many people. They are durable, easy to handle, etc.

For profound losses, they are almost a requirement since much more power can be used without forcing feedback (because of the greater distance between the microphone and earmold tip). Also, many assistive devices are designed for use with BTE aids, either through the T-coil or a boot which plugs into the aids.

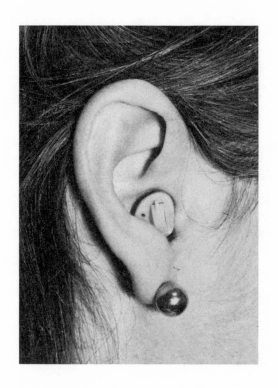

Canal Hearing Aid

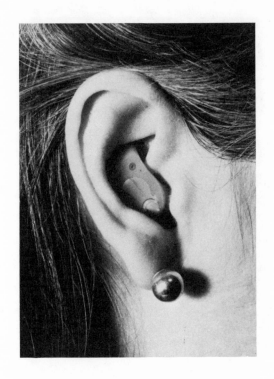

Low-profile Hearing Aids

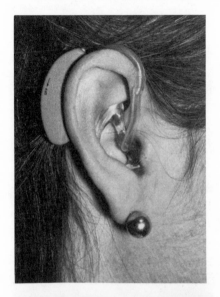

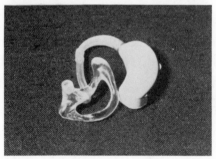

Behind-the-Ear Hearing Aid

Cros aids are used when one ear is weak and has no hearing at all. A microphone on that side picks up and transfers sounds to the good ear. This does not provide true stereophonic sound because one ear does all the hearing. It does avoid the problem of sounds on the off side becoming much weaker as they travel around the head to the good ear.

The connection to the good ear used to be through eyeglass frames or wires behind the head. Today, FM radio frequencies have been set aside for this purpose and wireless transmission is possible.

Bi Cros aids are used when the good ear is impaired and needs amplification. Otherwise, they are exactly the same as Cros aids.

Eyeglass aids. The hearing aid parts are enclosed in the earpieces (bows) of the glasses. Tubing connects the speaker outlets just in front of the ears to the earmolds.

This type of aid is rapidly disappearing because of problems with connecting the hearing aid bows to the wide variety of newer eyeglass frames and the length of time required to fit and care for them.

I suggest you avoid headaches by avoiding eyeglass aids if at all possible.

Body aids fasten to the front of your clothes and have a wire going up to a speaker which plugs into the earmold. They are now used mostly for profound losses. The mold tip is a long way from the earmold tip and much more power can be applied without causing feedback (see photo on page 137).

They are not very suitable for mild losses because of noise produced by cloth rubbing on the case. (Those with profound losses don't hear this noise.) Also, not

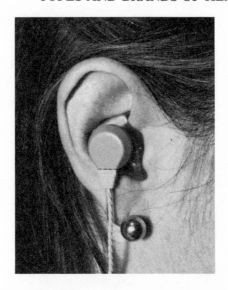

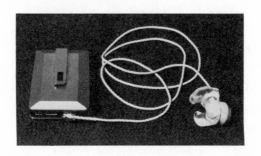

Body Hearing Aid

much is heard from behind, since the body blocks the sound.

Bone conductor aids operate by applying sound vibrations to the bones behind the ears.

Some sounds can be heard this way, but the understanding achieved is very poor compared to aids using earmolds. These aids are usually used only where there is no ear canal or when there is chronic canal drainage. Training in lip-reading is especially helpful when this type of aid is used.

Different Brands

Different brands and different models of the same brand have slightly different sounds. If your aids are being replaced, the new ones will of course sound unlike the old ones, but after a few days this should be no problem.

Today's aids emphasize high frequencies for better understanding. Even though they don't sound as *loud,* better *understanding* can be proved with a variety of tests. And understanding, not loudness, is why you want hearing aids.

T-Coils on Hearing Aids

T-coils pick up magnetic forces from *some* telephones and certain group listening systems or personal listeners. (See Chapter 16 on Assistive Devices.)

Most hearing aids are available with T-coils. The greatest use is in BTE aids for severely impaired people. To activate T-coils, a switch is moved to the T position and the volume nearly always turned higher as needed to pick up signals from magnetic loops, suitable phones, etc. *Be sure* you turn the volume down before returning the switch to the normal listening position.

So How Do You Decide Which?

I think it's usually best to do as dispensers suggest. They know your loss, the shape of your ear, and what has provided the best results for them in the past. If you are replacing aids, your brand preference may no longer be valid.

You probably can be a better judge of which dispenser rather than which type or brand. And success will depend far more on your willingness and effort than on any particular type or brand.

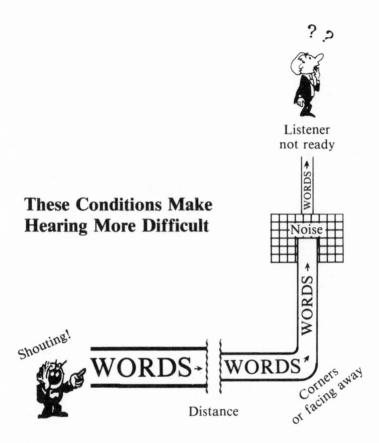

**These Conditions Make
Hearing More Difficult**

To improve listening conditions:

- **Don't shout**—it usually does **not** help.
- Instead, move **closer,** where it's **quieter,**
  where you can **face** each other.
- But even more important, begin with unimportant
  words so the listener is **focused** and **ready to listen.**

CHAPTER **21**

USING HEARING AIDS

The first step: the dispenser will make impressions of your ears. (Ears are as different as fingerprints.) These impressions are sent to a lab where earmolds or AIE aids are manufactured.

Earmolds or AIE Cases

Considerable experience and skill are required to make good ear impressions and the lab likewise. Comfortable earmolds or cases are absolutely necessary for successful hearing aid use. Don't try to use them if they hurt. They are hard, ears swell against them and get worse, not better.

For mild losses, some looseness is usually desirable to produce resonance for better sound quality. A good rule: no tighter than the degree of loss requires to prevent feedback.

If molds or aids aren't quite in place, the aids may hurt or fall off and be lost or damaged.

If drainage, swelling, or any sign of infection appears, stop wearing the aids and see your doctor. Some people are allergic to some molds or AIE cases. Non-allergenic materials are available.

Trial Periods

Make sure you don't waste your trial period. The dispenser needs your full cooperation. This means trying sincerely. When something doesn't seem right, go back and have it explained or fixed. Cooperate and communicate.

No matter how good the hearing aids, you'll still need to practice good listening habits.

Reviewing, you need:
- To be ready to listen.
- To face and be faced.
- Little background noise.
- To be near enough.
- To have time to "digest" the sounds and form words and thoughts.

Don't be in a hurry. Hearing aids are a major investment in money and in your future. You'll hear so much more at first, you may be tempted to buy the aids at once. Be careful. A trained voice close by in a quiet dispenser's office is not a good measure of what hearing aids will do elsewhere.

You need to try them in your *home* and your *life* most of your waking hours until you are sure.

Some people get along fine from the beginning, others have a discouraged period after the first glow of success. But stay with it and give them a real try.

Your first task will be putting the aids in place on

or in your ears. This will seem awkward at first, but with practice, you'll do it easily (you've learned to do far more difficult things in your life).

Volume Control Adjustment

Caution: Turning volume controls too loud may cause headache or dizziness for some people, especially when first wearing aids. Sometimes aids which do not protect against loud sounds can have a similar effect. Be careful.

With mild losses, I'm convinced proper volume control adjustment is the key to successful use of hearing aids. One of my greatest frustrations has been in not finding better ways of teaching this effectively.

Here's how aids end up in the dresser drawer when only one aid is worn. The volume is turned too loud to make up for both ears and fills the head with racket. In reaction, the volume is turned too low or off. Then it's worse than nothing because the ear is now plugged up. Realize the limitations of only one aid, or try a second.

Another way to fail: trying two aids at once without *any* plan or method for proper adjustment.

The volume should be as loud as possible without distorting background sounds. But, you say, "How will I know when the sounds are natural? I don't hear naturally." You learn to recognize the *break* between natural sounds and distortion.

Experiment with one aid first. Turn on a faucet and focus on the water sound as you turn the volume on your aid louder. You'll hear the sound getting louder and brighter until all at once it changes to a roar. It no

143

longer sounds like a faucet running—that's unnatural, distortion. Practice until you can set the aid just below the distortion—that's natural.

Try listening to your car. This fine machine which hummed like a sewing machine before now sounds like a cement mixer. Turn the volume up until you find the break into distortion and back till it's loud but natural. Like setting the idling jet on a carburetor, you must go too far and back in order to find the proper place.

Now try with your own voice. If this works, it is the best method, because your voice is always with you. Talk or hum and look for the place where your voice changes and begins sounding unnatural. This change may be pronounced or it may be very weak, but work on finding it. Then you'll be able to reset your aids as you talk *wherever* you are.

Don't try to adjust your aids for general use by using the TV. (You don't have any way of knowing how loud it actually is.) Not by a ticking clock either: the sound may be entirely out of the speech range. And, if you try to set according to another's voice, what happens when they aren't there? You need some method to set your aids according to the background noises around you.

> When you find a way to set your
> volume controls properly for *you,*
> wherever you are, most of your prob-
> lems with hearing aids will disappear.

For two aids, first set one, up and back, up and back, until it sounds right and leave it turned on (it won't interfere if it's properly set). Then adjust the other.

This often happens: You'll be comfortable with the sounds in quiet, but when you enter a noisy place, everything seems loud. In a restaurant, perhaps the newspaper crackles, the silverware clanks, the kitchen noises sound as if they were at your table. Unnatural sounds. Distortion. That means one, or both, of your aids are set too high. Adjust slightly till you are comfortable. And that's where best understanding *in noise* will occur.

Practice wherever you are. Up *too far* and *back,* over and over, several times a day. Practice in the quiet of your home, outside and in noisy places such as markets, too loud and back. Volume control setting gets easier until it's automatic for most people.

> We with mild losses must make peace
> with these volume controls or we won't
> like hearing aids.

You may hear comments like this: "You spent all that money for hearing aids, why don't you turn them louder so you *can* hear?" You'll soon learn that, with mild losses, turning louder makes understanding *worse* wherever there is background noise. (Of course, people with more severe losses *must* have them loud enough to understand at least for the times when they need to hear.)

If you still have trouble understanding after you've learned to adjust the volume controls properly, instead of turning them louder, go back to improving listening conditions.

Feedback

Feedback is a whistling sound which occurs when sound from the aid escapes back out of the ear and reenters the aid microphone, making a continuous round-trip. Some of the newer aids now have circuits which cancel out feedback.

Feedback may be normal for mild losses when you cup your hand around the aid. It will be more noticeable when a vent is required to fit your loss. (Vents are holes which allow certain sounds to escape back outside rather than reach the eardrum.)

With behind-the-ear aids, earhooks or tubings can crack, causing a peculiar high-pitched type of feedback. Since more power is necessary for severe losses, molds need to be tighter to prevent feedback. Molds must be replaced whenever they get so loose feedback occurs at the level needed for hearing. Causes of looseness: some materials shrink with age, we lose weight, our ears (and nose) grow all of our lives.

Hearing Aid Care

Hearing aids, like watches, usually stop when dropped on hard surfaces. At the beginning, practice putting them on and taking off over a carpet. Unlike most watches, aids are not waterproof. Wipe them with a dry tissue each night and more often during the day if needed before perspiration and skin oils can work their way inside and cause corrosion.

Once a week or whenever needed remove any ear-wax, etc., from the mold or case tip per directions with aid.

The tubings on BTE aids need to be changed whenever they turn yellow or get stiff—otherwise it may break off or pull out of the mold, causing the aid to be broken or lost. If water collects in these tubings, it can usually be removed by firmly grasping the aid with the earhook over your finger and shaking vigorously (like shaking down a thermometer). Do this over a carpet or bed, so it won't break if it gets away.

> Caution: Keep hair spray away from hearing aids. It gums up the volume controls and often means a factory reconditioning. Even the fumes alone can be harmful.

More don'ts:

- Don't use the new instant glues on your molds or aids (it freezes volume controls and dissolves some plastics).
- Don't use the volume control knobs to remove AIE aids (when one pops off you are out of business until after a repair job).
- Don't let dogs get your aids (they like to chew them—expensive).
- Don't wrap aids in tissue or paper towels to protect them (they may be thrown away).
- Don't leave aids behind when they have been removed to answer the phone.
- Don't leave batteries inside to corrode aids which aren't being used for extensive periods.

Batteries

Battery problems are the most frequent cause of hearing aid difficulties (weak, dead, wrong size). Here's a common trap: After resting overnight, batteries work fine for a short while then go dead without the user being aware. For many people, the first sign of a dead battery is a feeling of stuffiness.

Batteries aren't dated, so be careful where you buy them. Busy dispensers' offices are usually the best. *Be sure* to double check and get the proper size.

Some don'ts:

- Don't buy more than a 3-month supply at a time.
- Don't mix old batteries with new ones.
- Don't carry batteries loose—they will short out against each other or coins, etc. I learned this by burning a hole in my slacks only (lucky again).
- Don't try to make two batteries last the same length of time when wearing two aids. Either change them both when the first goes dead or each one as necessary.

There are many types and sizes:

- *Zinc-air* batteries are the newest and most widely used. The hold their voltage longer than mercury batteries. They last about twice as long and cost about twice as much. Don't remove the seal (on each battery) until you are ready to use the battery.

- *Mercury* batteries used to be the most common. Don't continue using them until they are completely dead because the sound quality will drop when the voltage gets too low.

CAUTION: Batteries Are Dangerous!

1. **Batteries can be harmful if swallowed.** Keep them in a safe place **away from children.** If batteries are swallowed get medical attention immediately. Hospital emergency rooms are often the quickest. Furnish them this number, (202) 625-3333 collect, so they can get information about battery contents, the latest treatment methods, etc.

2. **Batteries may leak or explode** if **recharged** or **burned.**

Hearing Aid Warranties

Manufacturer's warranties are usually for one or two years and are limited to reconditioning. Some companies extend their warranties for a small additional charge per year.

Repairs After the Warranty Period

Manufacturers make every effort to restore their aids to the original performance in order to protect the company name. They usually guarantee repairs for six months. Most will repair their aids for five or six years (longer if parts are available).

Don't expect hearing aids to last indefinitely. Your hearing changes and aids get better. Sometimes new aids are a better buy than repairs.

Insurance

Today, insurance is almost as important for hearing aids as it is for cars.

Hearing aids are expensive, small and fragile, easily dropped or lost. Pets are especially intrigued by the odor or sound and are likely to chew, hide or bury them. You'll feel much more comfortable buying and using hearing aids when you know they'll be insured.

One or more years of guaranteed repairs are usually included in the purchase price, but not for accidental damage or loss. Some household policies will insure hearing aids, usually at an extra cost, but proving losses can sometimes be a real problem.

Discuss all this with your dispenser.

Hearing aids are the finishing touch in your program for overcoming hearing loss problems. They are a "sound" investment in good living. Give them a sincere try.

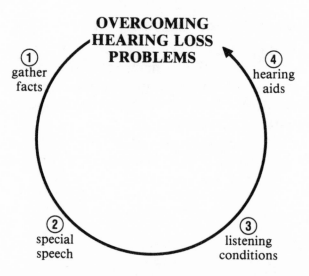

OVERCOMING HEARING LOSS PROBLEMS

① gather facts

② special speech

③ listening conditions

④ hearing aids

CHAPTER 22

PUTTING IT ALL TOGETHER

For **everyone,** hearing-impaired or not, who wants to **hear** and **be heard,** the rules seem to fall in "fours":

① Listening Conditions

1. Move closer.
2. Wait or move closer when it's noisy.
3. Avoid talking around corners or facing away.
4. Make sure listener is ready.

② Special Speech

1. Move closer.
2. Attract attention and face listener.
3. Speak slowly and distinctly.
4. Wait or move closer when it's noisy.

③ **Listen** and **try** to understand. When you can't, say exactly **why** in a clear, non-blaming manner.

④ Use all available technology: assistive devices, hearing aids, whatever **you** can find to make your life better.

And now the end . . .

All right, that's what I'd like to have known about hearing loss many years ago. If I had, surely my life would have been very different today. (And I very likely wouldn't have written this book.)

If you are as hardheaded as I am about learning, you'll benefit by going over this book again and again. Each time your viewpoint will have changed and you'll pick up new ideas for improving your life.

In another generation, perhaps recognizing early hearing loss and using special speech will be household knowledge. *You* can have a part in making this happen. First, pass this book around. Talk it up and make a difference in *your* neighborhood. Ask your library to order copies. Ask your bookstore to stock it.

Next, write and tell me what you like and dislike, what's interesting and what's boring, what was clear and what wasn't. This will make the next revision that much better.

Thank *you* for "hearing" me out.

Alec Combs
c/o Alpenglow Press
P.O. Box 1841
Santa Maria, CA 93456

APPENDIX

ORGANIZATIONS

These organizations supply help and information free unless otherwise noted. Toll-free phone numbers only are shown. TTY service is available as noted (call information for current numbers).

Academy of Dispensing Audiologists ADA
900 Des Moines St., Suite 200, Des Moines, IA 50309
Telephone: (515) 266-2189

Alexander Graham Bell Association for the Deaf
Nonprofit, membership. Mostly for children, but some services for adults. TTY.
3417 Volta Place, N.W.
Washington, DC 20007

American Association for Retired Persons (AARP)
Nonprofit, membership (for people 50 or over). Recent focus is on reducing medical costs. $5.00 annual fee includes subscription to *Modern Maturity* magazine, reduced-rate pharmacy, insurance, etc.—a bargain. Booklet, "Have You Heard?" free to members (see bibliography following).
1909 K Street, N.W.
Washington, DC 20049

American Speech-Language-Hearing Association
(National Association for Hearing and Speech Action)
Literature and referral lists. Voice and TTY 800-638-8255

10801 Rockville Pike
Rockville, MD 20852

Better Hearing Institute
Nonprofit, educational. For a list of hearing care professionals in your area, call Voice 800-424-8576. TTY.
1430 K Street, N.W., Suite 600
Washington, DC 20005

Food and Drug Administration
Federal agency, several publications about hearing and
hearing aids.
    8757 Georgia Avenue
    Silver Spring, MD 20910

Hearing Industries' Association
Represents companies who make or distribute hearing aids.
Literature.

    1800 M Street, N.W.
    Washington, DC 20036

National Association of the Deaf
Nonprofit, membership, literature, referral lists.

    814 Thayer Avenue
    Silver Spring, MD 20910

National Hearing Aid Society
    Has a Hearing Aid Help Line for consumer
    information about hearing aids, hearing loss or
    hearing health care.
        800-521-5247
        20361 Middlebelt
        Livonia, MI 48152

National Information Center on Deafness
Information, research, TTY

    Gallaudet College
    800 Florida Avenue, N.E.
    Washington, DC 20002

Self-Help for Hard of Hearing People, Inc. (SHHH)
Membership, chapters nationwide. Magazine, pamphlets,
extensive literature (small cost). See page 113 of this book.

    7800 Wisconsin Avenue
    Bethesda, MD 20814

BIBLIOGRAPHY

(Prices change—write and they'll advise.)

Ears to Ya
Consumer Survival Kit $1.00

Maryland Center for Public Broadcasting
Owings Mill, MD 21117

Facts About Hearing and Hearing Aids
15-page pamphlet (1981). One copy free

Council of Better Business Bureaus, Inc.
1515 Wilson Boulevard
Arlington, VA 22209
(or call your local Better Business Bureau)

Facts About Hearing and Hearing Aids
31-page pamphlet (1978). $1.75
Order number SN 003-003-02024-9

Superintendent of Documents
U.S. Government Printing Office
Washington, DC 20402

Have You Heard?
Hearing Loss and Aging
Up-to-date information (1984)
Free to members of AARP (address and details in Appendix under Organizations).

Hearing Aids
NBS Monograph 117
Technical information. 55¢
Order number SN 003-003-00751-0

Superintendent of Documents
U.S. Government Printing Office
Washington, DC 20402

How to Buy a Hearing Aid
10-page article $1.00

> Reprints, *Consumer Reports*
> P.O. Box 1949
> Marion, OH 43305

Tuning in on Hearing Aids
8-page (1981) One copy free

> FDA—Office of Consumer Communications
> 5600 Fishers Lane
> Rockville, MD 29857

**Special Devices for Hard of Hearing, Deaf,
and Deaf-Blind Persons**
297 pages, very thorough but becoming dated. (1981)
$14.95

> Little, Brown and Company
> 34 Beacon Street
> Boston, MA 02106

As you can see, a great deal has been written about hearing aids, but very little about living with mild hearing loss.

GLOSSARY

Air-bone gap—occurs when puretones are heard louder through the bone behind the ear rather than through the eardrum. Indicates conductive hearing loss (a problem in the middle ear).

Assistive device—any device other than hearing aids used for helping hearing-impaired people.

Audiogram—a graph used by hearing-care professionals to represent hearing levels. See drawing on page 42.

Audiologist—a person trained to measure various aspects of hearing, to assist and rehabilitate hearing-impaired persons, etc. May also dispense hearing aids. Requires at least a master's degree and extensive training.

Audio loop—a "loop" of cable around the neck, under the carpet, around a room, etc., for producing magnetic forces which hearing aid T-coils convert back to audible sounds.

Binaural hearing aids—hearing aids worn on both ears.

BiCros hearing aids—are used when one ear is nonfunctioning *and* the good ear needs amplification. Otherwise, they are exactly the same as Cros aids (see below).

Bone conductor hearing aids—used when the ear canal is closed or drainage is severe. Sounds are heard (rather poorly) through the bone behind the ear.

Bone hearing level—part of a hearing test: indicates how well puretones (see below) are heard through the bone behind the ear.

Brainstem testing—measures hearing sensitivity without requiring responses from patients (enables testing of the very young).

CC (close-captioned)—this symbol appearing on TV programs means the broadcast includes a signal which produces words on the TV screen. Requires a CC converter.

Cochlea—part of the inner ear (see drawing on page 28).

Cochlear implants—implants intended to replace part or all of the function of the inner ear.

Conductive hearing loss—caused by something wrong in the outer or middle ear.

Cros hearing aids—sound is transmitted from a microphone on a nonfunctioning ear to the hearing ear.

Decibel—a measure of loudness (see drawing on page 42).

Discomfort level—part of a hearing test: the level at which puretones and/or speech becomes uncomfortable.

Discrimination—part of a hearing test: the percentage of a certain word list understood. May be tested with or without background noise.

Distortion break—the level at which sounds become unnatural as hearing aids are turned louder. See pages 143 and 144.

Earwax—a natural secretion in the outer ear. See page 26.

Feedback—a noise produced when the output of an amplifying system is loud enough to enter the amplifier's microphone. See page 146 for hearing aid feedback.

Frequency (or pitch)—cycles per second (Hertz). See drawing on page 41.

Hair cells—part of the inner ear. See drawing on page 28.

Hearing aid evaluation—a measure of how well hearing aids perform.

Hearing evaluation—a complete hearing test.

Hearing threshold—part of a hearing test.

Hertz—frequency, cycles per second.

High frequency—as related to hearing: the upper part of the hearing range. See drawing on page 42.

Impedance testing—measures air pressure in the middle ear and the ability of the middle ear to conduct sound.

Implants (cochlear)—implants intended to replace part or all of the function of the inner ear.

Important others—those people whose relationships are important to a hearing-impaired person.

Key words—words which must be heard in order to understand.

Lip (or speech) reading—''seeing'' part of words on the speaker's lips. More on page 45.

Maskers (tinnitus)—a device which introduces sounds into the ear in attempting to mask noises inside the head. More on page 37.

Medical evaluations—as related to hearing, this means doing examinations and tests to learn as much as possible about a patient's hearing loss.

Middle ear—the air-filled space between the eardrum and the inner ear. Contains the three smallest bones in the body. See drawing on page 28.

Mild hearing loss—an indefinite term, often used to describe conditions in which vowels are heard well and consonants are not. See drawing on page 42.

Moderate hearing loss—an indefinite term indicating a hearing level in the middle ranges of the audiogram. See drawing on page 42.

Nerve loss (sensory-neural)—a term more common in years past to differentiate inner-ear problems from those in the middle ear (conductive hearing loss).

Normal conversation—an indefinite term: depends on the speaker's voice strength and the nature of the words used (high or low frequency). See drawing on page 42.

Normal hearing—varies widely, especially with age. See drawing on page 42.

Not-hearing habits—habits that form slowly as the hearing weakens. Usually very difficult to change once acquired.

Otolaryngologist—a medical doctor who treats ears and throat.

Otologist—a doctor who treats ears.

Otorhinolaryngologist—a medical doctor who treats ears, nose and throat (ENT).

Otosclerosis—a type of conductive hearing loss caused when the tiny bones of the middle ear no longer transmit sound properly from the eardrum to the inner ear.

Pitch— our perception of frequencies. See drawings on pages 41 and 42.

Presbycusis—a hereditary type of sensory-neural hearing loss that comes with aging. More on page 30.

Profound hearing loss—almost all ability to hear is missing. This is a severe handicap, requiring speech-reading training, extreme hearing aid amplification, assistive devices, etc. See drawing on page 42.

Projection (voice)—speaking in a way that makes the voice stronger, carries farther and of course is easier to understand. See page 86.

Puretone—a sound composed of only one frequency. Used in hearing tests.

Puretone hearing threshold—a part of a hearing test. A puretone for each frequency is presented through an earphone and the loudness gradually adjusted until the puretone is barely heard. This level is marked at each frequency one ear at a time and points then are connected (see the heavy lines on the audiogram drawing, page 42).

Severe hearing loss—commonly used to mean losses of 60 to 90 db.

Special speech—used in this book to mean speaking in ways which help hearing-impaired people understand. More in Chapter 13 (page 83).

T-coil—part of a hearing aid that picks up magnetic forces generated by audio loops, certain phone amplifiers, etc., and converts these forces back to normal sounds.

T-switches—activate T-coils.

Tinnitus—means hissing, ringing, buzzing or clicking noises inside the head. It can be devastating. More on page 37.

Tinnitus maskers—a device which introduces sounds into the ear in attempts to mask noises inside the head. More on page 37.

Trigger words—words which divert our thoughts, causing us to stop listening. More on page 71.

TTY phone devices—words are typed into one of these devices, converted to phone signals which are printed as words again on a receiving TTY machine. Then the process is reversed, and so on, back and forth.

Tympanic membrane—another name for the eardrum.

Volume—loudness measured in decibels.

White noise—a noise, such as running water, which masks all speech sounds.

ILLUSTRATIONS

INDEX

INDEX

S

Self-Help for Hard of Hearing
People 113
Sensory-neural hearing loss 28
Severe losses 18, 86, 132
SHHH 112
Signalling devices 102
Signs of mild loss 55
Sound waves 39, 41
Special speech 17, 83, 84, 85,
118
• and practice 86
• and severe losses 86
• and uncertainty 87
Speech (lip) reading 31, 45, 49
Stress 53, 54
Strong low frequency sounds
43
Strong voices 43
Sudden hearing changes 33

T

Tape recorders 105, 111
T-coils 105, 132, 138
"Teacher Effectiveness Training" 69
T-switch 105, 132, 138
TDD phone devices 29
Telephone 29, 36, 102, 103
• amplifier 102, 105
• answering devices 106
• listening devices 102
Television 106
• listening devices 106, 107,
108, 109

Theaters 97
Tinnitus 35, 37, 38
• maskers 37
• workshops 38, 105
Trial periods 142
Trigger words 71
TTY phone devices 29
Tubings (BTE aids) 147
Tympanic membrane 29
Types of hearing aids 130

U

Uncertainty 51, 83, 85, 87
Unrealistic expectations 121
Used hearing aids 125
Using hearing aids 141
Usual terms 124

V

Verbal language 70
Vibrators (bed) 29
Voice magazine 112
Volume (decibel loudness) 40,
42
Volume control adjustment
144, 145, 146
Vowels 43

W

Warning signs 55
Warranties (hearing aid) 150
Water noise 47
Wax buildup 25, 33
Weak high frequency sounds
43, 83

X

Y

Zee...end.

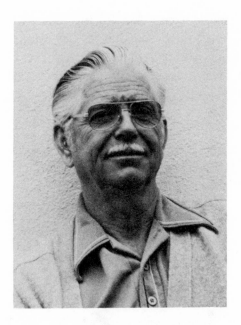

Alec Combs grew up on a small dryland Wyoming farm (wrinkle-belly country) during the depression.

He went to a small one-room school through the eighth grade, high school at Wheatland, Wyoming, then a degree in pharmacy at the University of Colorado.

He worked in an old-fashioned corner drug store for many years. He owned a drug store for 14 years and after selling it, worked as a hospital pharmacist. He sold his first hearing aids in one of these drug stores in the early '50s; later owned and operated two hearing aid offices until retiring recently.

He has four children, all college graduates, now scattered from coast-to-coast.

He has hunted, fished and travelled much of western

North America from Alaska and the Northwest Territories to Mazatlan; learned to fly at age 48; studied photography under Ansel Adams. He has completed most of the classes required for a Master's in psychology.

He says:

"I've lived a long and busy life. I've experienced many situations and places,
and enjoyed many fine people—I am indeed a fortunate man."

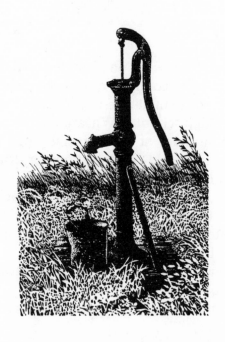

ORDER FORM

Alpenglow Press
Box 1841-B
Santa Maria, CA 93456

Please send me:

_____ copies of *Hearing Loss Help* @ $12.95 each.
                                ($14.95 Canada)

I understand that I may return this book in new condition for a full refund if not satisfied.

Name: _____

Address: _____

City: _____ State: _____ Zip: _____

Shipping and handling $1.50
      (total $14.45).

Californians: Please add 78¢ sales tax
      (total ($15.23).

☐ I can't wait 3 to 4 weeks for Book Rate.
   Enclosed is $2.50 for Air Mail shipment.

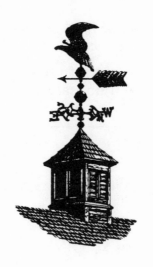

ORDER FORM

Alpenglow Press
Box 1841-B
Santa Maria, CA 93456

Please send me:

_____ copies of *Hearing Loss Help* @ $12.95 each.
($14.95 Canada)

I understand that I may return this book in new condition for a full refund if not satisfied.

Name: _____

Address: _____

City: _____ State: _____ Zip: _____

Shipping and handling $1.50
    (total $14.45).

Californians: Please add 78¢ sales tax
    (total ($15.23).

☐ I can't wait 3 to 4 weeks for Book Rate.
    Enclosed is $2.50 for Air Mail shipment.